Sally Hornsey runs Plush Folly, a leading cosmetics training company specialising in a range of cosmetic-making workshops, home study courses and kits. Awarded with Registered CPD Presenter status, Sally writes and delivers the workshops and oversees the home study programmes. She has taught many students how to design a range of bar and liquid soaps for their own use and has given them the skills and knowledge they need to establish a flourishing business. Plush Folly products have been sold in France, Germany and Luxembourg, and have graced the shelves of many shops, including Harrods and Fortnum & Mason, as well as appearing at the Chelsea Flower Show. Sally is also the author of *Make Your Own Perfume* and *Make Your Own Skin Care Products*.

Also by Sally Hornsey

Make Your Own Perfume
How to create your own fragrances to suit mood, character and lifestyle

Make Your Own Skin Care Products
How to create a range of nourishing and hydrating skin care products

How to Make Your Own Soap

in traditional bars, liquid or cream

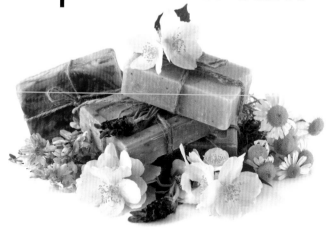

Sally Hornsey

Constable & Robinson Ltd
55–56 Russell Square
London WC1B 4HP

www.constablerobinson.com

First published in the UK by How to Books,
an imprint of Constable & Robinson, 2014

The material contained in this book is set out in good faith for general guidance and no liability can be accepted for loss or expense incurred as a result of relying in particular circumstances on statements made in the book. Those with allergies, or pregnant women, should take particular care when handling some of the ingredients used in soap making and, if in doubt should, consult a qualified medical practitioner.

A copy of the British Library Cataloguing in Publication Data
is available from the British Library

ISBN: 978-1-90897-423-5 (paperback)
ISBN: 978-1-84528-562-3 (ebook)

1 3 5 7 9 10 8 6 4 2

Printed and bound in the EU

This book is dedicated to the boys in my household
– Nick, Harry and Jonah, the best soap testers ever!

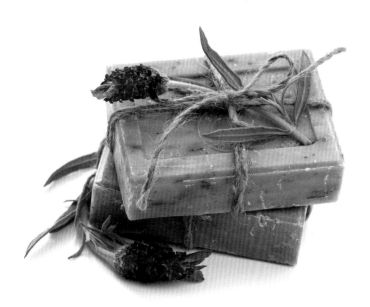

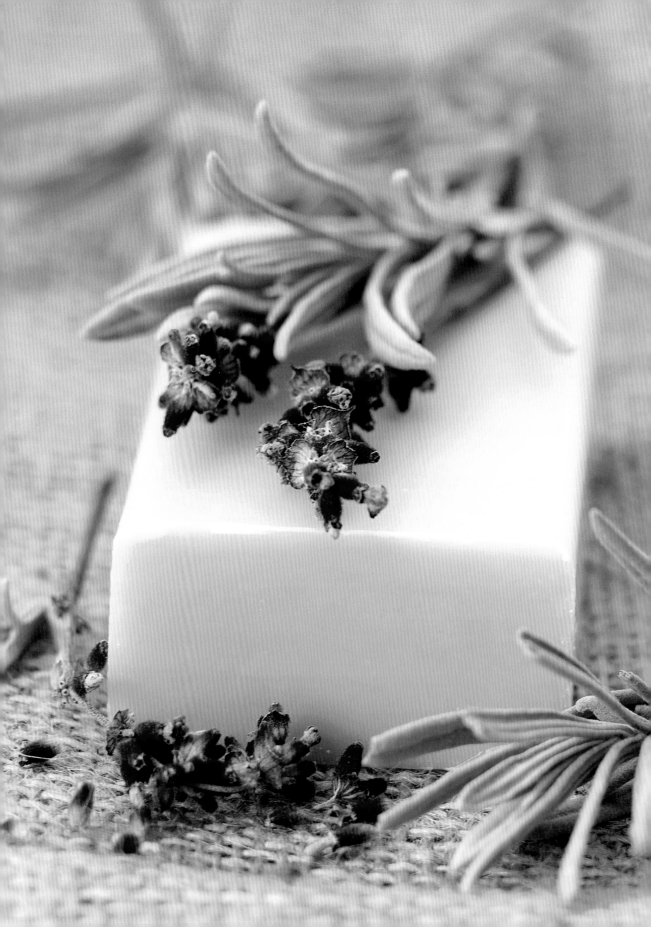

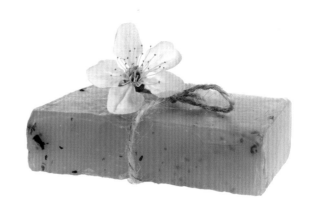

Contents

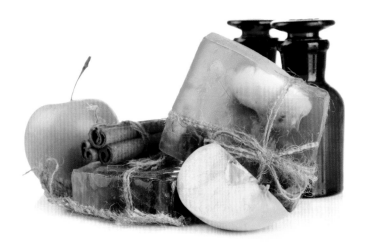

Acknowledgements

A giant thank you to everyone who helped me with various aspects of this book. To my lovely team at Plush Folly, who protected me from the phone, emails and visitors during the book writing and soap making sessions: you are all massively appreciated. Your next task is to help me use up all this soap . . .

The photographs in this book have been a labour of love and I thank Tom Weller and Chloe Strike for snapping away whilst I made soap. The biggest thanks of all go to Lizzi Roche, ex Plush Folly, who spent hours and hours with me, taking thousands of photos so that we could pick and choose the most appropriate ones for the book. Lizzi, you are a star!

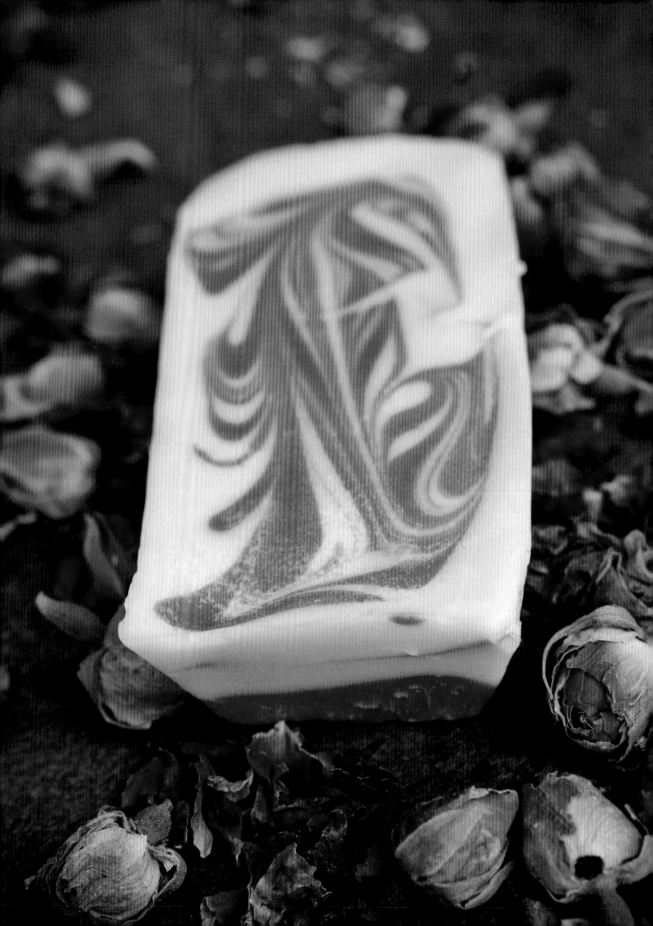

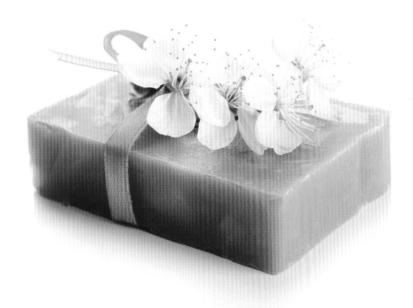

Introduction

Welcome to the world of soap making! If you have never made soap before, you are in for a real treat and I'm certain it won't take long before your soap making becomes a passion and addiction, even an obsession.

How to Make Your Own Soap covers a range of different soap types. I have included hard bars of soap and liquid soaps, bars crafted from pre-made bases and bars made from scratch, including making your own melt-and-pour base. The book also covers making liquid and cream soap using lye, as well as making liquid soap from surfactants.

It won't take long for you to discover that the biggest section in the book is the one on making hard bars of 'lye' soap, since it is here that you can experiment beyond your wildest imagination once you get the hang of making the soap. There are so many different ingredients that you can include in your soap, some of them quite surprising.

We have experience of soaps that include rain water, sea water, champagne, double cream, cow dung, rendered fat from road kill, stinging nettles, silk fibres, Halloween carved pumpkin leftovers, and even (forgive me here) excess fat from liposuction.

Handmade soaps can be beautiful to look at, as well as beneficial to the skin

This book covers techniques and methods to make an assortment of soaps and guides you through how to create your own versions of both hard bar and liquid soaps. I've tried to keep the recipe sizes small so that you don't start building too much of a soap mountain, but I'm certain you'll have plenty of friends and family willing to take excess soap off your hands. All the recipes can be doubled and multiplied upwards when you're ready to make in large quantities as the demand for your soap grows.

No matter what style of soap you are making, you will be dealing with hot liquids and possibly caustic ingredients too. Do take heed when handling these and make sure you follow all the safety precautions outlined in this book and on the ingredient packaging.

Enjoy your soap making adventure, have fun experimenting with the huge choice of ingredients available and relish how very, very lovely your soaps and skin feel when bathing.

CHAPTER ONE

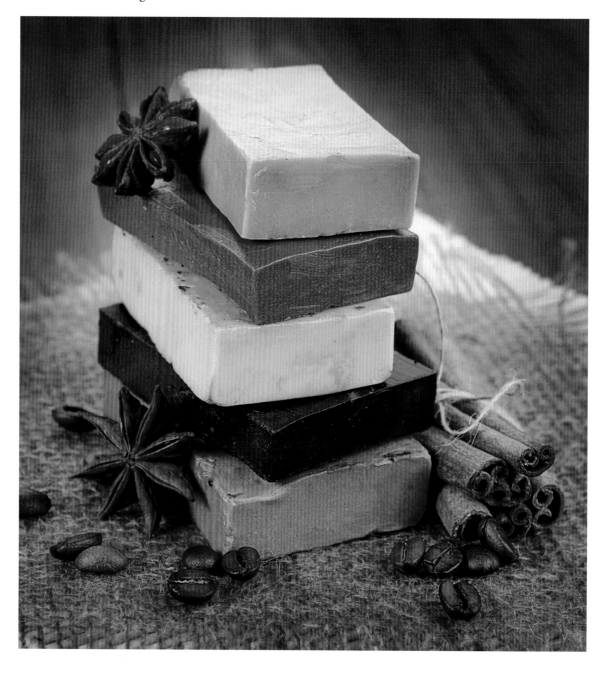

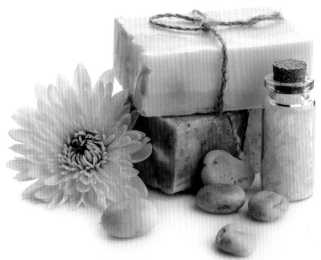

Making traditional bars of soap

Traditional soap is generally considered to be 'proper' soap. Rather than being created from a ready-made soap base, such as the melt-and-pour glycerine soap base, this type of soap is made from scratch using sodium hydroxide (also known as caustic soda), water and fats.

Traditional soap is made by combining a sodium hydroxide and water solution (also known as lye) with fats (natural oils, butters and waxes). The combination of

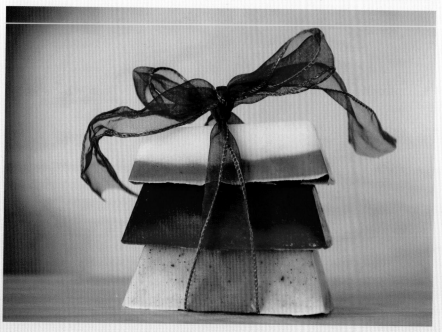

Beautiful handmade soaps

three basic ingredients – water, sodium hydroxide and fat – causes a chemical process called saponification, which results in the creation of hard bars of nourishing, lather-rich, moisturising soap.

There is no lye left in the final soap provided it has been made correctly.

Equipment needed to make traditional soap

Soap making uses similar equipment to cooking and whilst you may want to use your everyday saucepans and utensils, I strongly advise buying a set that you keep exclusively for soap making.

You can make soap on any type of hob – gas, electric, induction or aga – in a stainless steel saucepan.

The equipment you will need includes:

Saucepan
If you plan to make soap on the hob then you will need a heatproof container, such as a saucepan. The saucepan *must* be made of stainless steel to avoid any unwanted reaction with the lye.

Spoons
You will need a collection of stainless steel teaspoons, dessert spoons and serving spoons for stirring and dispensing ingredients.

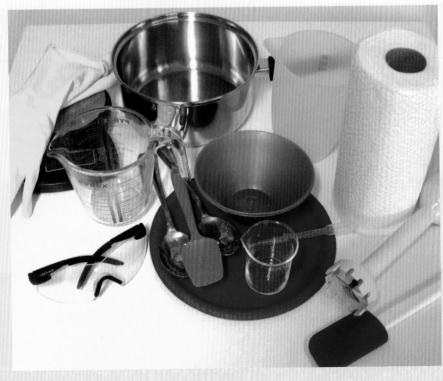

Basic equipment needed for making soap

Spatula
Use a long handled spatula for scraping any soap residue from the sides of the pan and jugs. Silicone spatulas are particularly flexible and can withstand the heat of the soap mixture.

Jugs and bowls
You will need a heatproof jug or bowl in which to mix and rest your lye solution. Whilst these can be made of thick plastic, they will deteriorate after many months of soap making so heatproof glass is better.

Digital scales
A set of digital scales is essential for accurate measuring of your ingredients. *Never* guess the weight as the recipe can go wrong and the soap can be potentially dangerous if the measurements are not precise.

A handheld stick blender
This is such a useful piece of equipment – every soap maker should have one in his or her toolbox! Whilst it is possible to make soap without a handheld stick blender, it will save hours of stirring if you use one.

Moulds (with or without mould liner and something to fix the liner in place)
Once your soap is ready it will need to be poured into your chosen moulds. Some moulds may require lining to make it easier to remove the finished soap, in which case you may need pegs or tape to hold the liner in place.

Old towels and blankets
If you are using the cold-process method, your soap will need to be insulated during the first 24 hours. To do so effectively, cover your soap with layers of blankets or towels.

Protective clothing
Although you don't need full overalls, at the very least you will need safety glasses, protective gloves and an apron. These will protect your skin, eyes and clothing from any unwanted caustic splashes.

Kitchen paper towels, cloths and hot water
Soap making can be very messy! Keep a roll of kitchen paper towels or cloths to hand to wipe up any spillages.

Sundry equipment
Depending on the method you choose to make your soap, you may also need a slow cooker (also known as a crock-pot) or an ovenproof container with lid.

SUITABLE MOULDS FOR SOAP MAKING

Since traditional soap is made in bars, you will need a mould in which to set your soap. This may be a large mould, in which case your soap will need to be cut into smaller bars, or you may wish to pour your soap into individual moulds.

Whether you wish to use a purpose-made soap mould or a household item that doubles up as a soap mould, there are many, many shapes and sizes to choose from.

USING A PURPOSE-MADE SOAP MOULD

Many soap making ingredient suppliers will have a range of soap moulds available. Before you spend your money, think about what size and shape of soap bar you wish to make and whether you want to do any specialist colouring techniques. Some moulds and shapes are far more suitable than others depending on what you are trying to achieve.

Loaf or log moulds

A loaf mould produces a long block of soap, which can then be cut into individual soap bar sized slices.

Tray or slab moulds (with or without inserts)

A tray mould is similar to a loaf mould in that it produces a large slab of soap.

Individual bar moulds – shaped or plain

Individual moulds, or trays of individual moulds, are especially useful if you want to have shaped soap.

The moulds come in a wide variety of shapes – from flowers, food, animals, cherubs and letters of the alphabet to moulds with embossed messages, which then appear embedded in or on your soap bars.

Wooden, log-style soap mould with a silicone liner

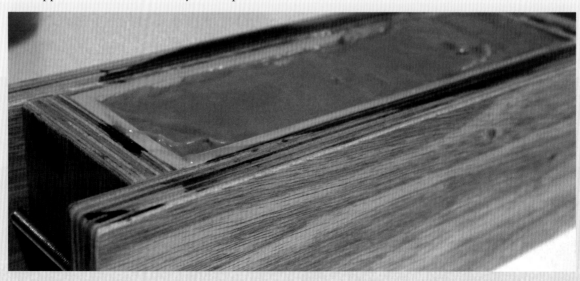

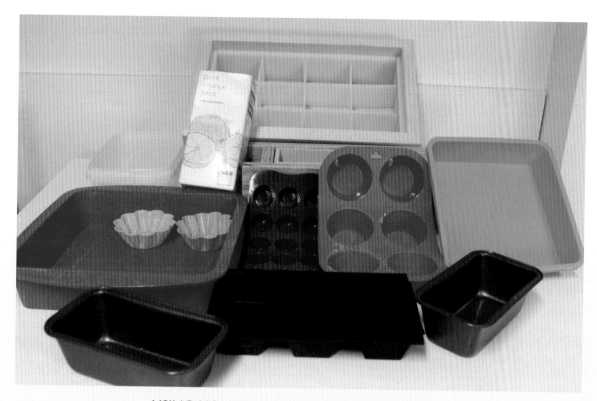

An assortment of soap moulds

USING HOUSEHOLD ITEMS AS SOAP MOULDS

It is at this point that I must apologise to you because from this moment on, you will always be on the lookout for everyday items that can double up as soap moulds. The shop assistants in my local supermarket have learnt to ignore me when I squeal with delight on finding an empty double cream carton holder on the dairy shelves to use in my soap making and my friends never even question now when I ask to keep a box or carton that they are about to throw away or recycle.

Forgive yourself the mould-searching obsession and just focus on the money you will be saving!

Juice or milk cartons

Rinse juice and milk cartons to remove traces of liquid. The top of the carton needs to be cut away to make it easier to pour in the soap mixture.

Mushroom cartons

I know it's more environmentally friendly to pack your mushrooms in paper bags but some supermarkets sell their very large mushrooms (suitable for stuffing) in long, plastic cartons. When washed, these make the most perfect log mould.

Shoe boxes

A shoe box is an ideal mould for a slab of soap. Please make sure you line it first with a waterproof lining such as clingflm to prevent the soap mixture from seeping into the cardboard.

Plastic ice cream tubs or lunch boxes

Any form of plastic box will double up as a soap mould. I was delighted when my children grew out of their school lunch boxes as I could then use these as soap moulds.

Cupcake or muffin cases

Paper cupcake and muffin cases are ideal for holding individual soaps. You may need to place these in a cupcake baking tin to support the sides of the cases.

Drainpipe

What better way of making a round soap than using a drainpipe? Any local DIY store will sell drainpipes and they may well cut them into shorter, more manageable lengths for you.

Whatever item you decide to use as a mould, always pour one test soap before pouring a whole batch – just in case the mould leaks, reacts badly to the hot soap mixture, or generally behaves in a way that you weren't expecting.

LINING YOUR SOAP MOULDS

Persuading your soap to pop out of the mould is a task in itself. The only moulds that I can guarantee the soaps will be easy to get out of are the silicone moulds. Lining your mould will make it much easier to remove the soap but, depending on the type of mould liner you use, it may not produce soap with super-smooth sides.

Moulds can be lined with parchment paper, greaseproof (baking) paper, freezer paper, waxed paper, cling film (also known as saran or plastic wrap) or polythene. If using parchment, greaseproof, freezer or waxed paper, line your mould as you would line a cake tin, holding the paper in place with a little masking tape. When using cling film or polythene, cut the lining material so that it overhangs the mould. Secure the lining in place with masking tape or by using pegs. You may be wondering if you can grease your mould in a similar way to greasing a bread tin. Alas, whilst this may work well for bread or pies, it won't do the same for soaps since the oily ingredient used to grease the mould is treated in the same way as the oil in your soap mixture and will be converted into soap. We have also tried to line our moulds with a liquid silicone such as cyclomethicone but have had no success here either.

REMOVING SOAP FROM THE MOULDS

If you have lined your mould, removing soap from the mould should be very easy. Note that the soap may still be a little caustic at this stage so you may wish to wear protective gloves when removing the soap from the mould. Simply turn the mould upside down over a flat, clean work surface and the soap should just release and gently fall from the mould. Carefully peel the liner away from the soap and discard the used lining.

If your soap is in a silicone mould, place the mould over a clean work surface and peel the mould away from the soap. The silicone mould can be washed in hot soapy water or in a dishwasher then used again.

If you have not lined your mould you will find it more difficult to remove the soap. Banging it onto the work surface and trying to pull out the sides of the mould may help, as will pushing down on the mould with the heel of your hand or thumbs, as if trying to release ice cubes from a tray.

I know soapers who put their soap in the freezer for a few hours to shrink the soap a little. Apparently the soap can then be eased or pushed out of the moulds but I haven't had much success with this method for traditional soap, although it works a treat for melt-and-pour soap that gets stuck in the mould.

If the soap is a little more stubborn and refuses to budge, you may have to exercise patience. As the soap cures, it hardens up and shrinks a little as it dries out. Soap that refuses to come out of the mould on day one may well be better behaved by week four and slip out of its mould easily.

Removing soap from a tray mould

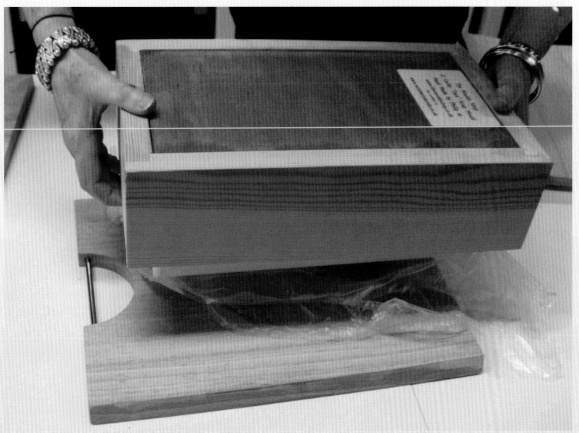

Soap is easy to remove from a silicone mould

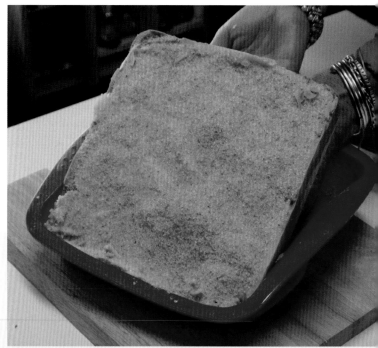

Choosing your soap making ingredients

You can use as little as three ingredients to make soap – water, sodium hydroxide and a fat. Whilst you have a choice of fats, there is no substitute for sodium hydroxide if you wish to make 'real' soap as this causes the chemical reaction that eventually converts the fats into soap.

SOAP MAKING INGREDIENTS – SODIUM AND POTASSIUM HYDROXIDE

Authentic, natural soap, both hard bar and liquid soap, is made from the chemical reaction of lye combined with fats. The lye is made from water (or water combined with other liquids) and an alkali. For hard bars of soap the alkali is sodium hydroxide, for liquid soaps the alkali is potassium hydroxide.

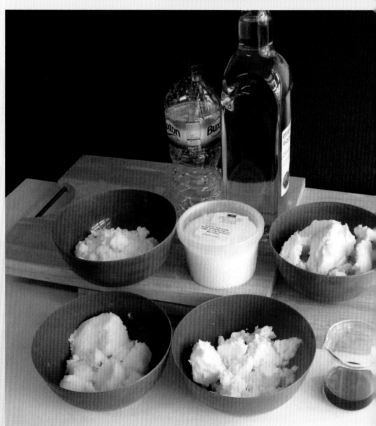

Prepare your ingredients before making your lye.

USING SODIUM HYDROXIDE

Sodium hydroxide is used for creating hard bars of soap. It is white and usually found in tiny granules – rather like very large grains of salt.

The chemical symbol for sodium hydroxide is NaOH (Na is sodium, OH is hydroxide). Sodium hydroxide is also known as caustic soda as well as being referred to by soap makers as lye.

USING POTASSIUM HYDROXIDE

Potassium hydroxide is used for creating liquid soap. It is usually found in hard flake form. Flakes are slightly off-white and sound like shards of broken porcelain when shaken.

The chemical symbol for potassium hydroxide is KOH (K is potassium, OH is hydroxide). Potassium hydroxide is also known as caustic potash as well as being referred to as lye.

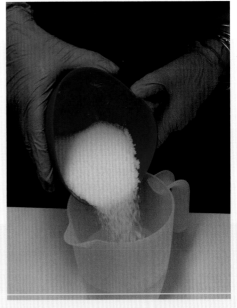

Sodium hydroxide mixed with water to create a lye solution

HANDLING THE SODIUM AND POTASSIUM HYDROXIDES

On no account should you touch the sodium hydroxide grains or potassium hydroxide flakes with your bare hands. *Always* wear safety gloves when handling these ingredients.

When mixing the sodium or potassium hydroxide and water to create your lye solution, you will find that the temperature of the solution increases as you stir. As it heats up, it will reach a temperature that causes it to evaporate as a steam and create airborne fumes. These fumes are unpleasant to breathe, so creating your lye solution should always be done in a well-ventilated room – make sure that the fumes are being blown away from rather than towards you.

HOW TO TREAT LYE SPLASHES

If you accidentally splash lye solution on yourself, rinse the affected skin under cold running water for at least 10 minutes. If your skin feels tingly, stings, burns, has blisters or concerns you in any way, seek prompt medical advice.

SAFETY EQUIPMENT REQUIRED WHEN MIXING SODIUM OR POTASSIUM LYE

It is absolutely essential that you wear protective gloves when handling lye. Household rubber gloves will suffice, but if you prefer something thinner and yet still as protective, nitrile gloves can be worn. Nitrile gloves are more resistant to chemical splashes than rubber gloves.

Make sure that your arms are covered when dealing with lye. As a sensible precaution, wear shoes, not sandals to prevent any splashes landing on your bare feet.

Since the lye may splash we strongly advise that you wear a pair of safety glasses. These are designed so that you can wear them over your normal spectacles, if necessary.

To prevent the lye splashing on your clothing, wear a protective apron.

If you feel that the fumes may be unpleasant for you, wear a protective mask to prevent breathing them in and make sure that you always work in a well-ventilated room.

As well as my recommendations, read and follow the safety guidelines on the sodium and potassium hydroxide containers. Soap making is not dangerous if you handle the sodium, potassium and other lye-associated ingredients correctly and sensibly.

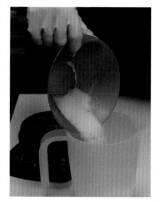

STORING SODIUM AND POTASSIUM HYDROXIDE

When not in use, keep unused hydroxides in their original containers. Store containers somewhere dry and cool, preferably at room temperature. Make sure the lid is securely fastened and keep containers out of reach of children and pets. If stored correctly, they have a shelf life of at least five years.

Always wear protective gloves when handling the lye ingredients

Label the containers correctly so that the contents can easily be identified as hazardous. Never store the sodium or potassium hydroxides in an unmarked container.

CLEANING SPILLED SODIUM OR POTASSIUM HYDROXIDE

If you spill sodium or potassium hydroxide granules or flakes, use an ash pan and brush to sweep up the spillage (be sure to wear safety gloves). Dispose of minor spillages in the sink and run cold water to dilute the hydroxide and flush it away. A regular plastic dustpan can also be fine as it will only melt if the solution is wet, in which case wipe up with disposable cloths while wearing safety gloves. If the spillage is large, consult your local authority about the best way to dispose of the waste.

Do remember that sodium hydroxide is sold as a drain cleaner, so disposing of it via the sink and the drain needn't be as harmful to the environment as you may think.

If you have spilt the caustic lye solution use thick kitchen paper towels to soak up the solution. Be sure to wear rubber gloves so that your hands do not come into direct contact with the solution. Place the paper towels in a polythene bag, tie the bag and then double bag it by placing in yet another bag before putting it in the bin.

Spray the area where the lye solution was spilled with vinegar as the acidic content helps to neutralise the alkaline in the lye. Leave for five minutes then wash the area with warm soapy water until you are sure there is no lye residue remaining.

SUPPLIERS OF SODIUM AND POTASSIUM HYDROXIDE

The hydroxides are available from specialist online cosmetic ingredient suppliers and you will find a list of these suppliers at the back of this book.

Since these ingredients are hazardous, they cannot be sent by Royal Mail post and will require transportation by specialist courier companies.

Sodium hydroxide can also be sourced from hardware stores since it is also sold as caustic soda, which is a common drain cleaning ingredient. Outlets such as Homebase, B&Q and Wilkinson in the UK may stock it. Just make sure that the container lists it as pure, or at least 97 per cent, sodium hydroxide rather than including it as part of a blend of ingredients.

HOW TO CREATE A LYE SOLUTION

Before you make up your sodium or potassium lye solution re-read the safety precautions and handling advice on the side of the container. Ensure you are wearing the correct protective clothing, such as safety glasses, gloves, an apron and a protective mask (optional).

Following the recipe carefully, weigh the cold water in a glass jug big enough to hold at least twice the amount of water needed for the recipe. Place the jug to one side so that it doesn't accidentally come into contact with the hydroxide before you are ready.

Measure out the sodium hydroxide (if making hard bars of soap) or potassium hydroxide (for liquid soap). If making cream soap you will need both sodium and potassium hydroxides. Weigh the hydroxide(s) into a clean, dry bowl. The bowl can be made of glass or plastic.

Add the measured sodium or potassium hydroxides to the water and stir gently to encourage the hydroxide to dissolve. Never add the water to the

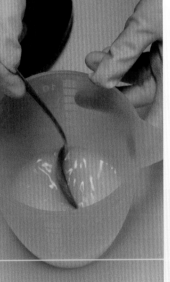

Lye solution mixed and ready for use

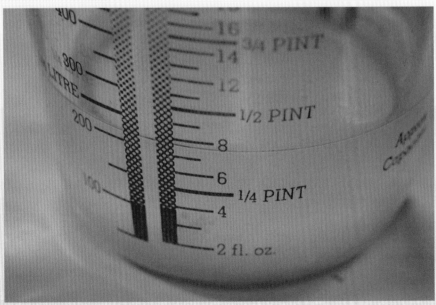

The lye solution will be hot and let off unpleasant fumes

hydroxide, always add the hydroxide to the water to start off as a very diluted mixture that gets stronger. Adding the water to the hydroxide would start with a very strong mixture that gets diluted – the first few droplets of water would make this too strong for regular handling.

Use a stainless steel, long-handled spoon to stir the mixture to avoid your hands getting too near the mixture.

Potassium hydroxide makes a whooshing sound rather like a steam train when it starts to dissolve. If you stir quietly, you should be able to hear it.

Keep stirring the lye mixture until you can no longer feel any un-dissolved particles of sodium or potassium hydroxide. This should take less than two minutes.

As the sodium or potassium hydroxide dissolves, the lye solution will become hotter, since the hydroxides are exothermic (the mixture will produce and let off heat). Once hot, it will start to release unpleasant steamy fumes, so always carry out the lye making in a well-ventilated room.

Set the lye solution aside somewhere whilst you get on with preparing your other soap making ingredients. Please make sure that whilst it is cooling, you leave it somewhere safely out of the reach of children and pets.

SOAP INGREDIENTS – WATER

There is a little choice when it comes to selecting your water. Since the water will be added to sodium hydroxide to create your lye solution, there is little point in using any specialist water, such as rose, frankincense or geranium hydrolats, as any active properties will be destroyed by the caustic element of the sodium hydroxide.

Most recipes will tell you to use spring or distilled water as part of your lye solution and I encourage you to follow this advice. Spring water can be easily purchased at supermarkets and distilled water may be found in the car accessories section of larger supermarkets or pharmacists. It is used to top up car batteries or to reduce the scale built up in kettles.

However, if spring or distilled water is not available, tap water will suffice.

Depending on where you live, your water may be hard or soft, and this can have a small impact on the lathering quality of bars of soap. I live on the London/Surrey borders and pretty much always use tap water for my soap making and have never noticed any adverse effect on the quality of my products. If you have a method of filtering and purifying rainwater, this can also be used as part of your soap making, as can seawater, although you may need to carefully select oils to ensure that your soaps are still able to produce lather.

Have fun experimenting with replacing some of the water with milks, fruit juices and other liquids. Refer to the section on substituting the water in your lye (page 86) to understand how to do this.

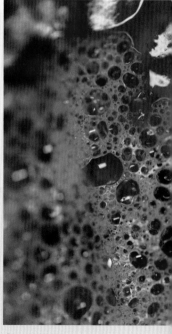

Coconut and castor oils will create a good lather

Basic fats, oils and butters needed to make soap

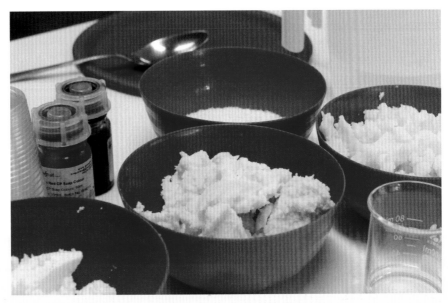

SOAP INGREDIENTS – FATS

Traditional soap was made by our very resourceful ancestors, who would have rendered down the bones and carcasses of chickens, pigs, cows and other animals and used the resulting fat as part of their soap making. Nowadays we are spoilt for choice, with a wonderful selection of luxurious and exotic oils and butters, all of which can be used in soap making.

Each oil, butter or wax brings slightly different properties to your soap. Some oils, such as coconut, will bring a quick, rich lather, whilst shea butter is richly moisturising and castor oil creates a fluffy lather as well as moisturising. Designing your soap by choosing different oils and butters is easy once you grasp some simple rules.

Fatty acids

You can use the fatty acid chart in the liquid soap section (page 137) to help you decide which oils to use, although some of the comments and benefits refer to how they will help liquid soap in a way which may not be relevant to hard bars of soap – for example, the coconut oil gives clarity to liquid soap but has no impact on the clarity of hard bars of soap as they will always be opaque. Beeswax helps to harden bars of soap but is unsuitable for use in liquid soap.

If you wish to use an oil or butter not included in this chart, use the internet as a research tool to find out what fatty acid content, iodine and SAP value individual oils have. The SAP value represents the amount of sodium or potassium hydroxide in milligrams required to saponify 1 g of oil or butter. The supplier's websites will often include this information, but if not, check the MSDS (Material Safety Data Sheet* overleaf) or certificate of analysis data sheets for a breakdown of the oil and butter components. These should be readily available from bulk cosmetic ingredient suppliers.

Iodine values

The lower the iodine value, the harder your bar of soap will be, so oils such as coconut, palm, palm kernel, cocoa butter and shea butter will produce harder bars than castor, sweet almond and avocado oils. Oils with iodine values of over 75 tend to make a soft soap, so team these up with a lower iodine value soap or include beeswax in your recipe to make a firmer soap.

PROPERTIES OF OILS, BUTTERS AND WAXES IN SOAP

Throughout this book I have highlighted any particular benefits that the oil will give your soap, but in terms of using the soap as a skin care product, since it is only on your skin for a matter of seconds before being rinsed off, it is unlikely that any major benefit will be acquired other than your skin will feel clean, soft, hydrated and lovely. The real beauty of the soap is in the feel of the sensuous, rich, creamy lather as you bathe, the beautiful aroma that wafts around your bath or shower awakening your senses, and the wonderful post-washing skin feel. If you plan to design your own soap, rather than follow an existing recipe, start by using the information below to decide which properties, and therefore which oils, you would like to use.

Fatty acid content of oils

Fatty acid	Cleansing	Conditioning	Fluffy lather	Stable, creamy lather	Hard Soap
Lauric acid	Yes	Yes		Yes	
Linoleic acid	Yes				
Linolenic acid	Yes				
Myristic acid	Yes	Yes		Yes	
Oleic acid	Yes				
Palmitic acid			Yes	Yes	
Ricinoleic acid	Yes	Yes	Yes		
Stearic acid			Yes	Yes	

Cleansing fatty acids

Oils that are rich in lauric and myristic acid are good cleansing bars. The soap molecules have the ability to attract the oils to the 'dirty' skin and hold onto them so that they cling to the soap and are rinsed away down the drain. Unfortunately they also remove precious skin oils so they can be drying if used in large proportions in your soap.

*Note: The Material Safety Data Sheet is a technical document containing all sorts of information, including how to store, handle and clear up any spilled ingredient, whether the ingredient is soluble, what form it is in, colour, texture and flash point and so on.

Conditioning fatty acids

Some oils will leave a little oily residue on the skin and help to moisturise and soften skin after the soap has been rinsed away. Choose oils rich in linoleic, linolenic, oleic and ricinoleic fatty acids for a soft, moisturised feeling after washing. Oils with a linolenic fatty acid content are mild and very suitable for sensitive skins. These oils are especially beneficial in hand soaps.

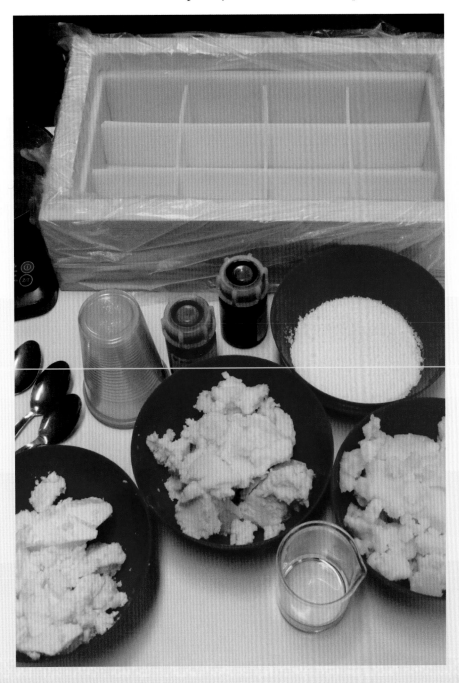

Soap making ingredients, equipment and mould set out ready to make soap

Fluffy lather fatty acids

Oils that are rich in lauric, myristic and ricinoleic fatty acids are quick to produce a quickly frothy, bubbly lather. Whilst the lather soon appears, it is thin and will dissipate fairly quickly, too.

Stable, creamy lather fatty acids

For a rich, creamy, dense lather that lasts a long time, choose oils with a high palmitic, stearic or ricinoleic content.

Hard soap fatty acids

If you are using oils with a high iodine value then you can counteract the potential softness of the bar by including an oil rich in lauric, myristic, palmitic or stearic fatty acids.

Oils, butters and waxes	Properties and approximate fatty acid % and iodine content	SAP value
Almond oil	Linoleic 18 Oleic 73 Palmitic 7 Stearic 2 Iodine value 100 A good all-round oil that is a useful addition to all soaps. It is naturally high in oleic acid to help give a lovely soft skin feel	0.137
Argan oil	Linoleic 35 Oleic 49 Palmitic 10 Stearic 6 Iodine value 99 A lovely conditioning oil but due to its cost, I recommend that you save your argan oil and use it as an additional superfatting oil rather than a substantial ingredient	0.134
Avocado oil	Linoleic 10 Oleic 62 Myristic 15 Palmitic 12 Stearic 1 Iodine value 90 Good for sensitive skins. Ultra-moisturising as it contains unsaponifiables which remain as oil rather than convert to soap	0.132

Beeswax	Beeswax can be used in soaps at up to 5 per cent of the weight of your oils. It may accelerate trace (page 38)	0.067
Castor oil	Linoleic 3 Oleic 7 Palmitic 2 Ricinoleic 87 Stearic 1 Iodine value 87 A must if you want a rich and quick-foaming soap. Castor oil acts as a humectant, helping to keep the skin hydrated after washing	0.127
Cherry kernel oil	Linoleic 41 Oleic 40 Palmitic 7 Stearic 2 Iodine value 126 Rich in linoleic and oleic acids, cherry kernel oil produces a conditioning bar. It needs to be blended with oils that can help to harden it up; on its own, it will produce quite a soft bar	0.138
Cocoa butter	Linoleic 2 Oleic 28 Palmitic 34 Stearic 35 Iodine value 38 Whilst the iodine value is low, if you make 100 per cent cocoa butter soap, it will be prone to becoming brittle and cracking. Keep the cocoa butter value to less than 20 per cent of your oil total	0.136
Coconut oil (semi-solid)	Lauric 54 Linoleic 2 Myristic 23 Oleic 8 Palmitic 8 Stearic 5 Iodine value 8 Up to 35 per cent coconut oil in your soaps makes a moisturising bar. Any more than that and it can become drying, courtesy of the high lauric acid content. Coconut oil produces a hard bar with a rich lather	0.180

Crambe seed oil (Abyssinian seed oil)	Linoleic 10 Oleic 18 Palmitic 3 Stearic 1 Iodine value 96 Crambe seed oil has a unique structure, making it very resistant to oxidisation. Team with oils that may deteriorate your soap (such as sunflower and safflower) to prolong freshness	
Grapeseed oil	Linoleic 68 Oleic 21 Palmitic 8 Stearic 3 Iodine value 130 Grapeseed oil conditions and softens the skin as it contains decent levels of linoleic and oleic acids. It produces a soft soap, so blend with oils that can make a harder bar	0.129
Hazelnut oil	Linoleic 9 Oleic 83 Palmitic 6 Stearic 2 Iodine value 97 Conditioning; be prepared for soaps with a high hazelnut content to take longer to reach trace (the point at which the oils and lye react with each other and start to convert the ingredients into soap – see page 38)	0.136
Jojoba oil	Linoleic 6 Myristic 1 Oleic 25 Palmitic 4 Stearic 45 Iodine value 83 Jojoba oil is a liquid wax and like beeswax, speeds up trace. It produces a rich, dense lather, but is not a particularly moisturising bar on its own. Use with other conditioning oils or as an additional superfatting oil	0.068

Lard	Linoleic 6	0.138
	Myristic 1	
	Oleic 48	
	Palmitic 32	
	Stearic 13	
	Iodine value 43	
	Lard soap gives a long-lasting, stable lather with good cleansing properties. Since lard is made up of animal fats, it is not suitable for vegetarians. However, it is cheap and easy to get hold of if you want to make your own soap and don't have access to more luxurious oils	
Mango butter	Linoleic 9	0.135
	Oleic 40	
	Palmitic 12	
	Stearic 45	
	Iodine value 60	
	Mango butter helps to harden up soap whilst bringing conditioning, moisturising properties to it. I recommend that you include it at 15 per cent of your oils	
Olive oil	Linoleic 10	0.134
	Linolenic 1	
	Oleic 74	
	Palmitic 11	
	Stearic 4	
	Iodine value 86	
	Virgin olive oil will do, but we tend to go for the rough and ready 'pomace' oil variety. Olive oil has a high oleic content and therefore makes an excellent skin conditioning soap. Soaps made with olive oil are mild but do not usually have an abundance of lather	
Palm oil	Linoleic 11	0.141
	Myristic 14	
	Oleic 40	
	Palmitic 30	
	Stearic 4	
	Iodine value 50	
	Palm oil produces a lovely, hard, waxy bar and behaves well in soaps. It will bring your soap mixture to trace fairly quickly	

Palm kernel oil	Lauric 46	0.155
	Oleic 18	
	Palmitic 8	
	Stearic 1	
	Palm kernel oil makes a very hard bar with a lovely, fluffy lather. Used at less than 35 per cent, palm oil is moisturising, but it can be drying at higher volumes	
Peach kernel oil	Linoleic 20	0.136
	Linolenic 1	
	Oleic 70	
	Palmitic 7	
	Stearic 2	
	Iodine value 115	
	Particularly good for sensitive skin, peach kernel produces a mild soap with a small amount of creamy lather	
Rice bran oil	Linoleic 38	0.129
	Oleic 48	
	Palmitic 11	
	Stearic 2	
	Iodine value 112	
	Rice bran produces a lovely conditioning soap that can leave your skin feeling soft and moisturised. It doesn't create a quick or long-lasting lather, so blend with other oils rich in palmitic or stearic acids	
Rosehip oil	Linoleic 50	0.133
	Linolenic 30	
	Oleic 13	
	Palmitic 3	
	Stearic 2	
	Iodine value 177	
	The gentle, healing properties of rosehip are lost if you use it to bulk out your soaps, so save this oil to use as an additional superfatting oil	
Safflower oil	Linoleic 65	0.135
	Oleic 30	
	Palmitic 4	
	Stearic 1	
	Iodine value 101	

High volumes of safflower will slow down both trace and curing times so I recommend that you use in combination with other oils, especially those that will make your soap harden faster

Shea butter	Linoleic 7	0.128
	Oleic 53	
	Palmitic 7	
	Stearic 43	
	Iodine value 62	
	Shea butter moisturises and nourishes the skin. It produces an ultra-creamy, moisturising bar, but being high in unsaponifiables, less than 100 per cent will convert into soap	
Sunflower oil	Linoleic 70	0.134
	Linolenic 1	
	Oleic 19	
	Palmitic 6	
	Stearic 4	
	Iodine value 127	
	Sunflower oil can deteriorate in your soap faster than other oils, so keep the proportions down and blend with other oils that have a high vitamin E content, such as avocado, wheatgerm or argan oil	
Wheatgerm oil	Linoleic 62	0.131
	Oleic 18	
	Palmitic 18	
	Stearic 2	
	Iodine value 130	
	Rich in antioxidant vitamin E, wheatgerm can be used in soaps to keep any shorter shelf-life oils fresher and prevent the soap from deteriorating	

Use this table to help you to devise combinations of your own. If you want a soap with a quick, fluffy and long-lasting lather to moisturise your skin, consider making a soap with coconut, castor and avocado oils with an added dollop of shea butter. But you will also need to take note of the column titled 'SAP value'. When making soap, it takes a defined quantity of sodium hydroxide to convert the fats into soap. Too much sodium hydroxide will make your soaps harsh and sting your skin (or worse) when you wash yourself. In contrast, too little sodium hydroxide makes your soaps oily and soft. The SAP value of a fatty acid indicates how much Sodium hydroxide you will need, so that at least 95 per cent of the oils, butters and waxes are converted into soap.

It is possible to calculate how much sodium hydroxide to use depending on your particular blend of oils, but for those of us not entirely comfortable with performing the calculations ourselves, there are plenty of tools available on the internet to do the maths for us.

CALCULATING HOW MUCH SODIUM HYDROXIDE TO USE IN YOUR SOAP

Unless you are gifted with the ability to perform mathematical functions, I suggest that you use a calculator to follow my example below. Remember, there are soap calculators on the internet that have been especially designed to work all this out for you and in reality, it is unlikely that you will ever do this manually. However, I do think you should understand why the calculations need be done and how you could do so manually should you ever be stranded, about to make your soap, but without internet access.

The purpose of the exercise is to work out how much sodium hydroxide you need to convert your chosen fats into soap. I have decided to use avocado, coconut, castor oil and shea butter as described earlier. As coconut can be a little drying, I've included this oil in a smaller quantity than the castor and avocado oils. Shea butter tends to be more expensive than the oils so I've included only a small amount as I'm on a budget.

The recipe I have designed for my 'moisturising with quick, fluffy and long-lasting lather soap' is as follows: 250 g castor oil; 200 g avocado oil; 100 g coconut oil; 50 g shea butter. That's 600 g oils in total.

The SAP value for each oil represents the amount of sodium hydroxide you will require per gram of ingredient in order to convert that particular ingredient into soap. For example, if I have 100 g of avocado oil whose SAP value is 0.132 then I would multiply 0.132 by 100 (grams) in order to gauge how much sodium hydroxide is needed to convert the 100 g avocado oil into soap. For my recipe, the calculations would be as follows:

Ingredient	SAP value	Maths formula	Sodium hydroxide quantity required
250 g castor oil	0.127	250 x 0.127 = 31.75	31.75
200 g avocado oil	0.132	200 x 0.132 = 26.4	26.4
100 g coconut oil	0.180	100 x 0.180 = 18	18.00
50 g shea butter	0.128	50 x 0.128 = 6.4	6.4
TOTAL			82.55

Therefore I can determine from my calculations that I require 82.55 g of sodium hydroxide to convert my chosen oils and shea butter into soap. If your scales do not measure in such small increments, rounding your sodium hydroxide down to 82.5 g (or even 82 g) is acceptable in the circumstances.

As each fat has its own SAP value, you cannot fiddle about with a recipe and swap one oil or butter for another without checking that the quantity of sodium hydroxide is still sufficient to convert the oils to soap. Failure to run it through a SAP calculator may result in a product that is too harsh for your skin or too oily and soft to be considered soap.

USING A SOAP CALCULATOR

There are many soap calculators available on the internet, all of which perform the same function but with a different interface. If you prefer to use an Excel spreadsheet, you can download your own soap calculator from the Plush Folly website. The calculator will also calculate your liquid soap and cream soap recipes too. If you prefer to enter your recipe details directly onto an internet site, the following soap calculators may be helpful:

www.plushfolly.com
www.thesage.com/calcs/lyecalc2.php
www.soapcalc.net/calc/soapcalcwp.asp
www.brambleberry.com/pages/Lye-Calculator.asp
xwww.cranberrylane.com/calculator.htm

CALCULATING HOW MUCH WATER TO USE IN YOUR SOAP

The last remaining calculation is to work out how much water I need to mix with my sodium hydroxide. Actually this bit isn't nearly as important as the sodium hydroxide calculation and if you are a bit over or slightly under, it won't matter. See the section on discounting the water in your soap for an explanation as to why this doesn't matter (page 131). The rule of thumb that we prefer to use is that *the weight of the water should be 37.5 per cent of the total weight of your oils.* My oils weigh 600 g in total so I need to work out 37.5 per cent of 600 g. To do so, I divide the weight of my oils by 100 (to get 1 per cent) and then multiply the answer by 37.5 (to get 37.5 per cent, which is the value of the weight of my water). The calculation would look like this: 600 / 100 = 66 x 37.5 = 225. For my recipe I would therefore require 225 g water.

That wasn't too bad, was it? But if you would rather be making soap than doing maths then forget everything you have just read in this section and use one of the online soap calculators to do all that for you. All you need to do is enter the weight of the oils you are using and the calculator will tell you how much sodium hydroxide and how much water you need to use.

Don't be too concerned if the soap calculator you use tells you a slightly different weight for the water: your soap will still turn out fine. Similarly, if your calculator is telling you a slightly lower weight of sodium hydroxide to use, that's probably fine too as long as it is only a small difference. Your calculator may be set with a superfatting default, which can change the sodium hydroxide quantity by up to 5 per cent. See the sections on water discount and superfatting for more information (page 130–1).

Fragrancing your soap

Having selected the oils and butters you want to use in your soap and having calculated the amount of sodium hydroxide and water, you will now need to make a decision on the aroma you wish to scent your soap with.

Both essential oils and cosmetic grade fragrance oils can be used to add a scent to your soap. If you wish to create a blend you can combine two or more essential oils, two or more fragrance oils and even combine essential oils with fragrance oils. Whatever smell you enjoy blending, you can probably include it in your soap. Do note that some fragrance oils may not behave as expected and can cause your soap to thicken very quickly.

The aroma of light and refreshing citrus essential oils, such as lemon, orange, lime, grapefruit, bergamot and mandarin, will fade far faster than richer aromas, such as patchouli and vetiver. You can buy extra-strength citrus essential oils, known as 5-fold or 10-fold, which will give your soaps an extra citrus burst. These are only suitable for soaps, since they are five or ten times stronger in aroma than regular essential oils.

Herbaceous aromas, such as rosemary, basil, eucalyptus, peppermint and lemongrass, hold their scent well in soap.

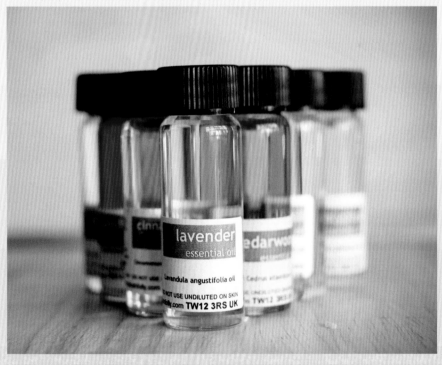

A selection of essential oils to fragrance handmade soap

THE DIFFERENCE BETWEEN ESSENTIAL OILS AND FRAGRANCE OILS

Essential oils are oils extracted from part of a plant. Different parts of the plant may yield a different aroma and all aromatic parts of the plant are used to make essential oils. Essential oils can be obtained from seeds, bark, petals, fruit peel, leaves, twigs, resins, berries, bulbs and roots, and are extracted most often by steam distillation, but may also be pressed, or extracted with a solvent. Essential oils are natural oils and are very potent.

Fragrance oils are manmade oils. They can contain components from an essential oil blended with synthetic aromas, or may be made up entirely of synthetic compounds. The manufacture of cosmetic grade fragrance oils in the EU is governed by a body called IFRA (International Fragrance Association). In the EU countries any fragrance oil that is sold as safe for use in cosmetics has to be IFRA approved. Essential oils do not come under the watchful eye of IFRA and can be used safely in cosmetics, provided you keep to the recommended usage rates.

USING FRAGRANCE OILS IN YOUR SOAP

Fragrance oils contain a blend of compounds that can work beautifully in your soap or may cause it to seize. Seizing is when your soap mixture goes from being a runny batter-like liquid to a very thick mixture that is difficult to stir and even harder to get into the mould. Seized soap is still safe to use but it may not be very attractive.

If your fragrance oil supplier is unable to tell you whether or not the oil will work in your soap, you will have to test it yourself. Take approximately 100 g of the soap batter and add 2 g fragrance oil to it. If you can stir the scented batter without it becoming too thick, then it is unlikely the fragrance oil will have an adverse effect on your larger batches. If, however, the smaller soap quantity has thickened up and has almost become solid, then it is best to choose a different fragrance oil for your soap.

REDUCING THE CHANCES OF SOAP SEIZING

If you wish to use a fragrance oil that you know will cause your soap to seize, there are a few techniques you can try that might reduce the speed at which the soap will seize, hopefully giving you plenty of time to get it into the mould before it starts to harden.

Firstly, make sure that your lye and oils are cooler than 35°C/95°F before combining them and mixing to a light trace (still runny). Adding the fragrance oils to a cooler soap batter may slow down the seizing.

Alternatively, reserve some liquid oil, such as olive oil, from the soap recipe and blend your fragrance oil into the reserved oil. For every 10 g fragrance oil, use 30 g reserved oil. Bring your mixture to a light trace and then add the fragrance oil and the olive oil blends and stir thoroughly into the soapy batter.

And finally you could try adding the fragrance oil to the melted warmed soap oils before combining them with the lye.

With any of the techniques suggested above, I recommend you work quickly just in case the soap starts to seize anyway.

HOW TO CALCULATE HOW MUCH FRAGRANCE OR ESSENTIAL OIL TO USE IN YOUR SOAP

You may be surprised at how much fragrance or essential oil is required in order to give your soap bars a good, strong, long-lasting scent. We fragrance our soap at 2 per cent, which initially gives a good aroma but fades a little from the outside edges of the bar as the soap ages. Once the soap is used in the bath or shower, the scent is reactivated and becomes more apparent.

For those wishing to have a stronger-smelling soap, it is possible to scent up to 5 per cent, but this may be too strong for some noses – and more importantly, too strong for sensitive skins. In order to calculate the percentage, you will have to add up the total weight of all the ingredients in your recipe excluding the sodium hydroxide. Once you have calculated the weight, divide it by 100 to get 1 per cent and multiply the result by 2 (to get 2 per cent) or up to 5 (to get 5 per cent). Using our 'moisturising with quick, fluffy and long-lasting lather soap' recipe the essential oil calculation would be performed as follows:

250 g castor oil
200 g avocado oil
100 g coconut oil
50 g shea butter
225 g water
82 g sodium hydroxide
TOTAL (excluding the sodium hydroxide) is 825 g

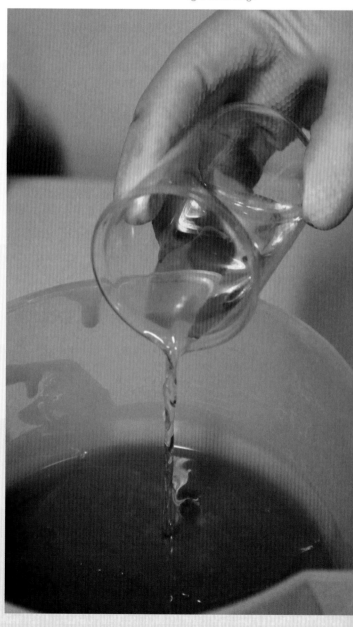

The fragrance or essential oils are usually added at the light trace stage

Now divide 825 g by 100 = 8.25 g so the value of 1 per cent is 8.25 g. If I wish to fragrance at 2 per cent, I will need to multiply 8.25 g by 2 (8.25 × 2 = 16.5) so I would require 16.25 g of fragrence oil. If I wish to fragrance at 5 per cent, I must multiply the 8.25 g by 5 (8.25 × 5 = 41.25) so I would require 41.25 g of fragrance or essential oil. Now you can understand why I said that you might be surprised at how much you need to use. I would suggest that you start with 2 per cent and decide whether this is strong enough once the soap has had a chance to mature.

Colouring your soap

Your soap will pick up its natural colour from the different oils you use and this is likely to be a pale beige to ivory shade. However, if you have used an orange unrefined palm oil, or a green unrefined avocado oil then your soap bars will have an orange or green tinge to them.

There are many natural ingredients that you can add to give your soap a colour and there are some manmade colours that you can use too. Be aware that your soap will be alkali and an alkali environment can cause some surprising colour changes, so you may not achieve the colour you expect.

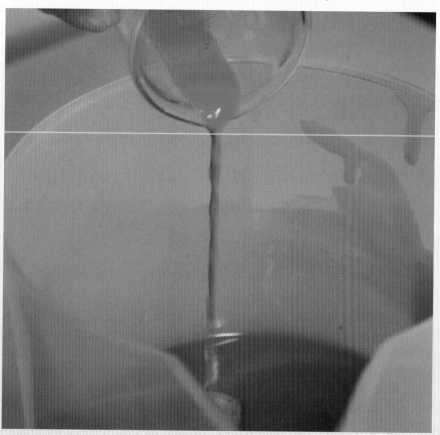

Some colours are not stable in lye soap and may change to a surprising hue

NATURAL COLOURING INGREDIENTS

Natural colouring ingredients that you can use in your soaps
include the following:

Ingredient	Colour in final bar	How to include in your soaps
Alkanet root	Pinkish purple	Infuse pieces of root in carrier oil (such as olive oil) and use the filtered pink carrier oil as part of your soap making oils, or add powdered alkanet root to your traced soap
Annatto seeds	Yellowish orange	Infuse seeds in carrier oil and use the filtered carrier oil as part of your soap making oils
Carrots	Pale to golden orange	Infuse grated carrot in carrier oil and use the filtered carrier oil as part of your soap making oils or substitute some of the water with infused carrot water
Cinnamon	Pinkish brown	Add cinnamon powder to traced soap mixture. **Warning**: this may be irritating to sensitive skin
Cocoa powder or plain chocolate	Brown	Add cocoa powder or melted chocolate to your traced soap mixture
Coffee	Brown	Add instant coffee granules dissolved in a little hot water to your traced mixture or add wet ground coffee orts (the waste matter after making ground or percolated coffee) to your traced soap mixture. The ground coffee makes an exfoliating bar
Cosmetic clays	Green, pink, red, yellow – there are many different coloured clays available	Mix with a little water and add to traced soap mixture
Madder root	Pinkish red	Infuse root in carrier oil and use the filtered carrier oil as part of your soap making oils or add powdered madder at trace
Paprika	Reddish brown	Add paprika powder to traced soap mixture. **Warning**: this may be irritating to sensitive skin
Spinach powder	Olive green	Add powdered spinach powder to traced soap mixture
Spirulina powder	Turquoise green	Add spirulina powder to traced soap mixture
Turmeric	Gold to yellow	Add turmeric to traced soap mixture. **Warning**: this may be irritating to sensitive skin

Do be prepared for the colours acquired using dried herbs and spices in your soaps to fade over time. Set a couple of random bars aside for at least six months, checking on the strength and stability of the colour during this time. Certain colours fade quickly, others less so.

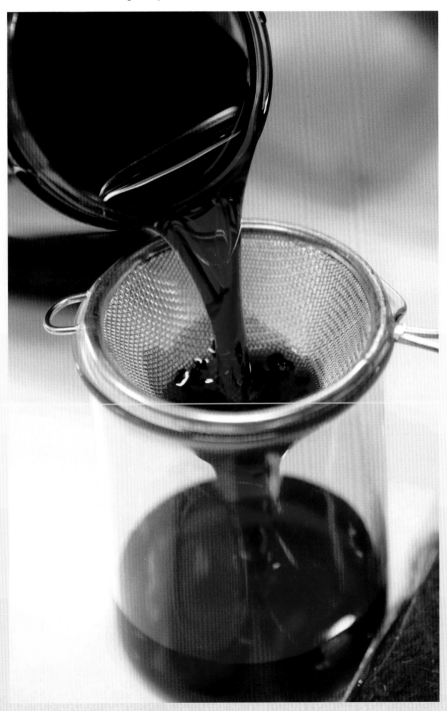

Olive oil infused with alkanaet root will add a purplish shade to the soap

USING COSMETIC GRADE COLOURS

There are a number of different types of cosmetic colour that can successfully be used in your soaps.

Type of colour	Comments
Dyes	Dyes are usually water-soluble and the powder variety will happily disperse in your traced soap mixture. Liquid dyes are already dissolved in water, alcohol, oils or glycerine. The common liquid colours purchased for melt-and-pour soap making are not stable in cold processed soaps and may well morph into a different colour – have fun experimenting!
Pigments (ultramarines and oxides)	Pigments are powdered colour that disperses either in water or oil. Mostly stable in cold processed soaps, they will not change colour although they may fade over time. To ensure a smooth colour block rather than speckles, blend the powders with a little warm water or oil before adding to your lightly traced soap mixture.
Lakes	Lakes are pigments and dyes that have been bonded onto a substrate such as sodium, potassium, alumina hydrate, zirconium or calcium strontium, which makes it insoluble. If a colour is insoluble it will not dissolve in water or bleed into other colours but still gives the appearance of a coloured soap.
Mica	Micas are beautiful metallic colours used to provide a shimmer, sheen and shine. They shimmer beautifully in transparent melt-and-pour soaps, but will lose their sheen in opaque cold process soaps, although they retain their colour. Add micas to lightly traced soap mixture.

HOW MUCH COLOUR TO USE

How much colour you add depends on whether you wish to colour the whole block of soap that you are making, or just part of it and if you want a tint of colour or quite a strong effect.

Each colour has a different strength. Using one teaspoon of liquid blue would give you a far stronger colour than one teaspoon of ultramarine. I suggest that you start with a small amount of colour, mix it into the soap well and add more colour if necessary until you have reached the desired shade.

Never add too much colour as this may result in coloured flannels, towels and the need to clean your bath, basin or shower after use. The bubbles and foam should always remain white.

As some colours can be unpredictable in your soap, consider testing a small amount of mixture first (see opposite) to avoid the finished result coming out differently from how you expected it.

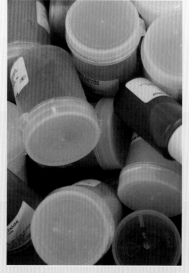

Oxide colours add muted earth tones to your soaps

TESTING YOUR COLOURS

Mix a small amount of soap to test the colour reliability

In order to determine the colour's stability in an alkali environment, perform a simple test before using it for the first time.

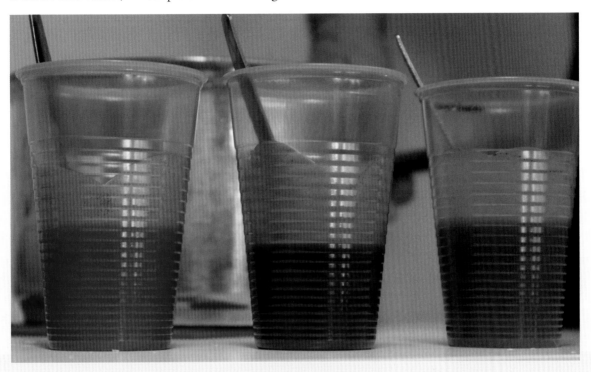

TESTING THE IMPACT OF THE LYE ON YOUR COLOUR

Make up a small amount of lye solution (5 g sodium hydroxide to 18 g water), ensuring that you adhere to all the safety precautions. Once the lye solution is cool, add a small amount of the colour you wish to test. Add either a few drops of liquid colour or a slurry of powdered colour blended in water or oil to the lye; mix the lye and colour together well.

Leave the coloured mixture somewhere safe for up to 24 hours to see what, if any, colour changes take place.

TESTING THE COLOUR OF THE FINAL SOAP MIXTURE

The most through and decisive test to see if a colour will work well in your soap is to take a small amount of the soap mixture out of the saucepan once you have reached light trace (still runny) and added a fragrance or essential oil.

Stir a small amount of your chosen colour into the soap mixture – preferably blended in oil or water first – and set the sample aside for 24 hours. Note any colour changes that take place.

WHAT HAPPENS IF A COLOUR ISN'T STABLE?

The alkali in traditional soaps may cause unexpected colour changes. I remember my first experience of this happening was when I decided to make some 'Lavender's Blue Dilly Dilly' soap, but had run out of my preferred blue colouring: ultramarine blue. Instead I decided to use the liquid blue colouring that I use in melt-and-pour soaps and bath fizz, also known as CI42090 liquid blue colouring.

Different colours and colour effects in soap

As I stirred the blue into the traced soap mixture it quickly changed from blue to a shade of grey, which wasn't what I wanted. I carried on as usual and poured the soap into the mould, covered it with layers of towels and blankets and left it for 24 hours.

You can imagine my surprise the next day when I took the soap out of the mould. Instead of having grey (or blue) soap, I had beautiful pink soap! We renamed the soap 'Lavender's Pink Dilly Dilly' and from that point on always made it with the liquid blue. The recipe is included later in this section (page 42) if you wish to try it for yourself.

Pouring purple colour into the saucepan

But that was a good luck story and we can't promise that you'll be excited by the colour changing results each time. Many of the brightly coloured natural ingredients, such as beetroot powder or grape skin powder, will turn a disappointing shade of brown, whilst manganese violet fades to brown and prussian blue is an instant brown.

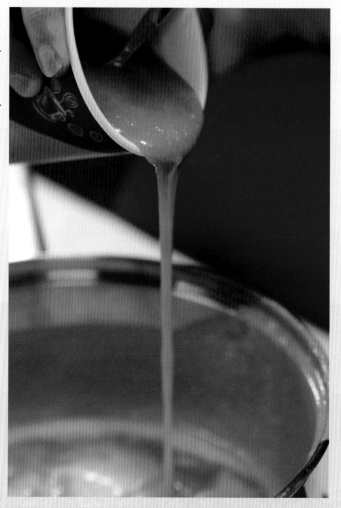

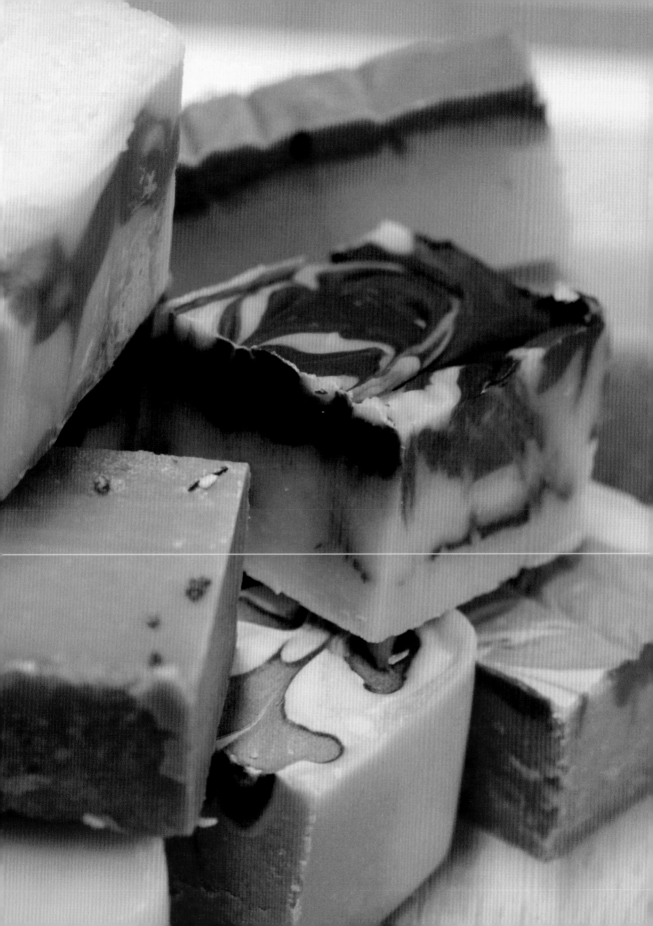

Soap making methods

So now that you have an idea of what oils, butters, colours and fragrances you would like to use to make your soap, and what moulds you are going to use to set your soap in, you now need to discover how to make the soap itself.

There are several methods of making bars of traditional soap and there are advantages and disadvantages to each of these different techniques, as detailed below.

COLD PROCESS SOAP MAKING

Although this is called 'cold' process there may be some requirement for heat. The heat is needed to melt any solid fats, such as shea butter, palm oil and beeswax, before they can be combined with the sodium hydroxide and water solution (lye). The lye solution itself will be hot, since it is exothermic and heats spontaneously – this is a natural reaction that occurs when mixing water and sodium hydroxide.

Whilst this might be a quick method of making soap, the soap then needs to rest for up to four weeks before it can be used. Although safe to use as early as two weeks, it will be on the soft side and more prone to going squishy when used. Cold process soap is often referred to as 'CP' soap.

NO HEAT METHOD

This is the quickest and easiest soap making method of all, but is only suitable once you are confident in handling the lye. It can only be carried out if you are using liquid or a very soft oil such as coconut oil. With this method, the liquid and soft oils are placed in a heatproof container and the naturally hot lye is poured over the top of them. The mixture can then be continued as cold process soap or heated using one of the hot process methods below. In the hotter summer months, many of the harder oils soften up naturally, making the no-heat soap making process even simpler.

HOT PROCESS SOAP MAKING

The hot process soap making method requires heating the cold process soap mixture in a pan over heat until the soap is cooked. This is more time consuming but the soap is ready to use as soon as it has hardened up (usually two or three days after the date of manufacture). Hot process soap is often referred to as 'HP' soap.

MAKING SOAP IN A SLOW COOKER (CROCK-POT)

The technique for making soap in a slow cooker is very similar to the hot

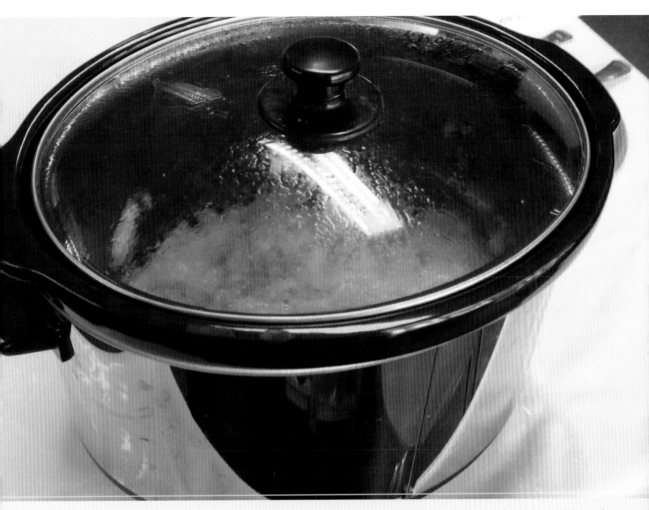

You can make hard bars and liquid soap in a slow cooker (crock-pot)

process soap making method, but very little intervention by you is required. This is ideal for those who don't wish to hang around stirring their soap mixture as it cooks. The cooked soap mixture is transferred to moulds and the soap is ready for use as soon as it has hardened up.

Soap made in this way is often referred to as 'CPHP', which stands for crock-pot hot process soap.

MAKING SOAP IN AN OVEN

The technique for making soap in an oven is very similar to the slow cooker (crock-pot) soap making method, and again, very little intervention is required. In this case, the traced soap is placed in a large, ovenproof, lidded pot and left in a warm oven whilst it cooks. Again, the cooked soap mixture is placed in moulds and the soap is ready for use as soon as it has hardened up.

Soap made in this way is often referred to as 'OPHP' or 'HPOP', which stands for oven process hot process or hot process oven process soap.

Method	Advantages	Disadvantages
Cold process	This is a very quick method of preparing your soap It is easy to know when the soap is ready to be poured into the mould The soap is still runny when poured so it is easy to perform fancy colouring techniques	It takes four weeks or so for the soap to be ready for use Your fragrance may not be as strong as you wish, since some of the aroma is lost due to the heat the soap reaches during the gel phase
No heat	This is the fastest method of preparing your soap It is easy to know when the soap is ready to be poured into the mould The soap is still runny when poured so it is easy to perform fancy colouring techniques	Whilst dealing with cold oils, you will be handling hot lye, which is the lye at its most dangerous
Hot process	The soap is ready to use very soon after making it Your fragrance may hold up better in the finished soap, since it has been added when the soap is hot, but cooling down Colours that are unstable in an alkali environment fare better in hot soap recipes, since the colour can be added after the soap has cooked and is no longer alkaline	The soap takes about an hour longer to make than the cold process method Regular stirring is required This method is not as simple for novice soap makers since it isn't always easy to gauge when the soap is ready to transfer to moulds The soap is much thicker when pouring so fancy colouring techniques are more difficult. These can be made easier by adding a little extra hot water to the cooked soap to make it runnier You will need to work very fast to get the soap into the moulds once ready, so that it doesn't set in the pan itself The soap will be very hot when you are placing it in the moulds
Slow cooker (crock-pot)	The soap is ready to use very soon after making it Little effort is required once the soap mixture has traced	This method is not as simple for novice soap makers since it isn't always easy to gauge when the soap is ready to transfer to the moulds
Oven process	The soap is ready to use very soon after making it Little effort is required once the soap mixture has traced	This method is not as simple for novice soap makers since it isn't always easy to gauge when the soap is ready to transfer to the moulds

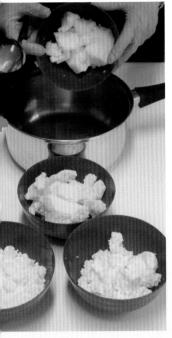

Basic soap recipes

If you're not quite ready to formulate your own recipes, then I have included several recipes that are relatively straightforward to start you off.

Each of the recipes yields approximately 600 g of soap mixture: enough for six 100 g bars or a large 600 g block of soap. If you don't have the fragrance or essential oils we have suggested, please feel free to substitute with your preferred scent blend or one from the blends section included in this book (page 24). For each recipe follow the steps below, which use the cold process method. See the individual recipe notes for any special instructions.

MAKING SOAP USING THE COLD PROCESS METHOD

There are ten easy stages for making cold process soap. I estimate that it will take about an hour from weighing the ingredients to covering your soap in towels unless you plan to do any fancy swirling or colouring techniques, in which case set aside a further 15–20 minutes to carry out the colouring part of the soap.

Step 5: Weighed oils and butters ready to add to the saucepan for melting

Step 1

Get all your equipment, ingredients, safety wear and sundries ready. Line your mould if necessary and place to one side.

Step 2

Weigh out the water required for the lye solution. Place the water jug to one side whilst you weigh your sodium hydroxide.

Step 3

Weigh your sodium hydroxide, making sure that you adhere to all the safety instructions given in the section about handling sodium hydroxide (page 9).

Step 4

Carefully tip the sodium hydroxide into the water and stir until there is no gritty feeling at the bottom of the jug, as this indicates that all the sodium hydroxide has dissolved.

Step 5

Weigh the oils, butters and waxes and transfer to a saucepan. Place on the heat until the solid oils, butters and waxes have melted. Do not include the essential or fragrance oils in this saucepan yet.

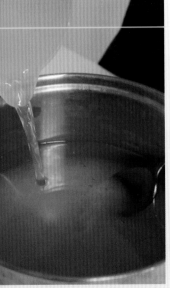

Step 6: Adding lye to the melted oils

Step 6

Wearing your safety goggles and gloves and paying careful attention to the safe handling of the lye, pour a very small amount of lye into the melted oils. If there is no reaction, such as the oils trying to fizz and react to the lye, carry on carefully pouring the lye into the melted oils.

Step 7

Stir the oils and lye together until they form a light trace (still runny). Whilst you can do this task by hand, you will find it much quicker to perform using a handheld stick blender. Blitz the soap mixture with the blender until it reaches trace. This will probably take about two or three minutes depending on the temperature of the oils, the ambient temperature and whether or not you have oils that may speed up or slow down reaching the trace stage.

Trace is when the soap mixture looks rather like a pancake batter or custard. When you drizzle a little of the soap batter back into the mixture it will briefly sit on the surface before sinking into the rest of the batter or when you can see a shape left by the blender when you lift it out. Light trace is when your batter is still runny, medium trace is slightly thicker soap batter and heavy trace is very thick soap mixture that will dollop rather than pour smoothly when you tip it out.

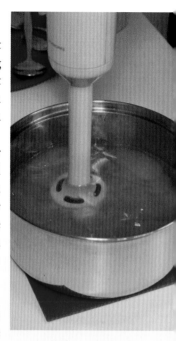

Step 8

Unless specified in the individual recipes add the essential or fragrance oil to the lightly traced soap batter and stir well. Stir right down to the bottom of the saucepan, so that fragrance or essential oils are thoroughly incorporated into all the soap mixture.

If you are adding colour or other additives to your soap, it is likely that they will be added at this step. Stir well after each addition.

Step 7: A stick blender will save you the time and trouble of mixing by hand

Step 9

Pour the soap mixture into your prepared mould.

Step 10

If the mould does not have a lid, cover with a chopping board or piece of cardboard to prevent the towels falling into the soap. Then cover the covered mould with a layer of old towels. The more the merrier as it's important that the soap is kept insulated for the next 24 hours.

There, that's it – all you need to do now is clear up, wash up and wait!

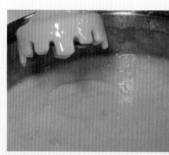

A light trace is where you can see a shape left in the soap from the blades of the stick blender

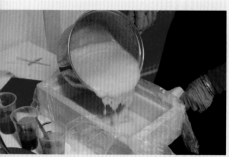

Step 9: Pouring soap into the mould

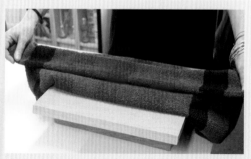

Step 10: Cover your soap with layers of towels or blankets for the first 24 hours

SOAP RECIPES USING THE COLD PROCESS METHOD

Cold process soaps are quick and easy to make once you get used to making and handling the lye and oils. The soap takes a few weeks to harden up before they can be used, but the wait is worth it since the result is skin-softening, moisturising, luxurious bars of soap that you'll love.

Slumber bar

The slumber bar is a gentle soap with delicious aromas of lavender and ylang ylang, both known for their ability to lull you into a state of relaxation. Use this soap for your pre-bedtime bath. Toss a handful of rose petals into your bath too just for the sheer beauty and opulence.

LYE SOLUTION
168 g water • 63 g sodium hydroxide

SOAP OILS AND BUTTERS
150 g olive oil • 100 g sweet almond oil • 100 g coconut oil
50 g avocado oil • 50 g mango butter

SOAP SCENT
3 g lavender essential oil • 11 g ylang ylang essential oil

METHOD
Follow the ten easy cold process soap making steps (pages 37–8).

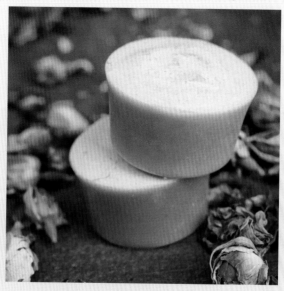

Slumber bar

Meek and mild

This soap is mild and gentle, courtesy of the oils high in linolenic acid, especially rosehip. To maximise the properties of the rosehip oil, it is added after light trace and with the essential oils, so don't accidentally add it to the saucepan with the other oils.

LYE SOLUTION
168 g water • 62 g sodium hydroxide

SOAP OILS AND BUTTERS
220 g olive oil • 150 g peach kernel oil • 40 g coconut oil
40 g palm oil • 20 g rosehip oil (add with the essential oils)

SOAP SCENT
10 g chamomile essential oil • 2 g lavender essential oil

METHOD
Follow steps 1–7 of the cold process soap making steps (pages 37–8), making sure that you do not include the rosehip oil with the other oils. Once you have reached a light trace, add the rosehip oil when you add the chamomile and lavender essential oils and continue with steps 9 and 10.

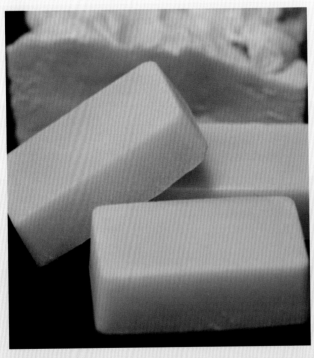

Meek and mild soap, courtesy of rosehip and other oils high in linolenic acid

Skin so soft

The shea butter and kukui nut oil make this a fabulous skin softening soap. The beeswax will harden the bar up as otherwise it tends to be initially on the soft side and may take longer to solidify. Beeswax will help to bring your soap to trace fairly quickly, so you may not need to use your handheld stick blender for as long as usual. I love to decorate this one with a rosebud or two.

LYE SOLUTION
148 g water (instead of making your lye with 168 g water, use 148 g water; the other 20 g will be used to make a milky solution, below)
56 g sodium hydroxide

SOAP OILS AND BUTTERS
130 g olive oil • 100 g castor oil • 100 g kukui nut oil
100 g shea butter • 20 g beeswax

SOAP SCENT
6 g lavender essential oil • 6 g rose geranium essential oil

ADDITIONS
15 g milk powder mixed with 20 g water (that you kept back when making the lye). If you warm the water first, the milk powder will dissolve more easily.

METHOD
Follow steps 1–7 of the cold process soap making steps (pages 37–8) until you have reached light trace. Add the milky solution with the lavender and rose geranium essential oils and continue to steps 9 and 10.

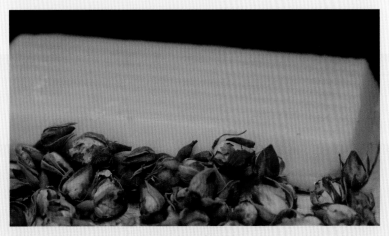

Skin so soft soap

Lavender's pink dilly dilly

This is the soap that went from blue to grey to pink (page 32), so don't be surprised when it starts changing colour in front of you! It won't be fully pink until you remove it from the mould after 24 hours.

LYE SOLUTION
168 g water • 63 g sodium hydroxide

SOAP OILS AND BUTTERS
220 g olive oil • 100 g coconut oil • 80 g palm oil • 50 g shea butter

SOAP SCENT
12 g lavender essential oil

COLOUR
A few drops of blue liquid colouring CI42090

METHOD
Follow the 10 easy cold process soap making steps (page 37–8) to recreate this soap, remembering to add a few drops of blue colouring after you have added the lavender essential oil. Once you have stirred the liquid blue colouring into the soap, it should start to change to a shade of grey whilst you continue to steps 9 and 10.

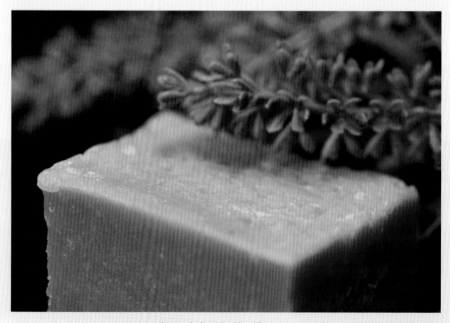

Lavender's pink dilly dilly soap

Citrus hit

This is an uplifting and refreshing aroma. If you don't have 5- or 10-fold lemon (extra strength), make a blend of lemon, lemongrass and may chang essential oils, as the citrus smell will last longer than if you had used lemon essential oil on its own.

LYE SOLUTION
158 g water (instead of making your lye with 168 g water, make it with 158 g water; the remaining 10 g will be used to make a slurry with the yellow oxide, as this causes the yellow colour to disperse more evenly)
62 g sodium hydroxide

SOAP OILS AND BUTTERS
200 g olive oil • 100 g sweet almond oil • 100 g coconut oil
50 g castor oil

SOAP SCENT
4 g lemon essential oil • 4 g lemongrass essential oil
4 g may chang essential oil

COLOUR
1 g yellow oxide
(mixed with the 10 g water that you kept back when making the lye)

METHOD
Follow steps 1–7 of the cold process soap making steps (pages 37–8) until you have reached light trace. Add the yellow oxide solution with the lemony essential oils and continue to steps 9 and 10.

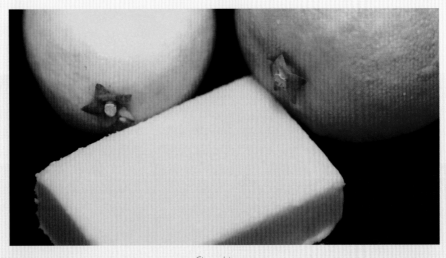

Citrus hit soap

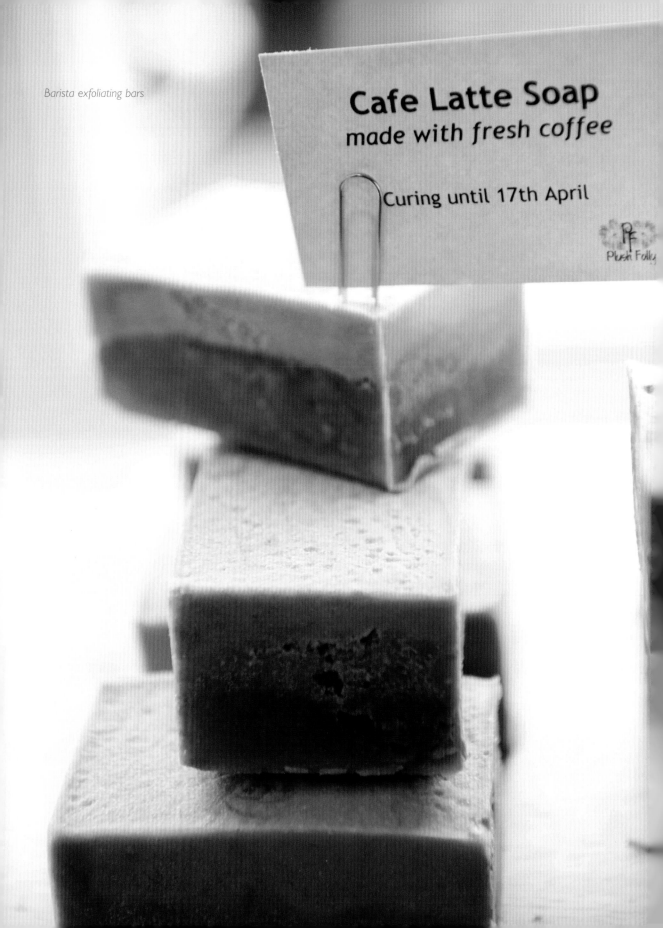

Barista exfoliating bars

Cafe Latte Soap
made with *fresh coffee*

Curing until 17th April

Plush Folly

Barista exfoliating bar

This is one of my favourite soaps! Save the leftover coffee grounds from your cafetière, as they are ideal for use in soap. They will give a natural brown colour and make your soap an exfoliating bar, since the grounds will go hard.

If you are feeling adventurous, split your soap mixture into two halves and add the coffee grounds to one half and the milk powder to the other. This allows you to have a bar of soap that is half exfoliating and half creamy, a colouring technique known as layering.

LYE SOLUTION
148 g water (instead of making your lye with 168 g water, make it
with 148 g water; the other 20 g will be used to make a milky
solution with the milk powder, below)
65 g sodium hydroxide

SOAP OILS AND BUTTERS
200 g olive oil • 150 g coconut oil • 50 g palm oil • 50 g shea butter

SOAP SCENT
12 g coffee fragrance oil

ADDITIONS
15 g milk powder mixed with the 20 g water that you kept back when making
the lye (warm the water first to make the milk powder disperse more easily)
20 g freshly ground coffee (or leftover coffee grounds)

METHOD
Follow steps 1–7 of the cold process soap making steps (pages 37–8) until you have reached light trace. Add the coffee fragrance oil and stir well.

Split the mixture into two halves by leaving one half in the saucepan and pouring the other into a jug. You don't need to be exact; guessing how much is half will work fine for this recipe.

Add the milk solution to one half and mix well. Add the coffee grounds to the other half of the soap mixture and mix well. Pour the coffee grounds half into the mould and spread the soap mixture with a spatula to fill the mould evenly. Slowly pour the creamy half over the darker coffee grounds half, being careful not to dislodge the darker coffee layer too much.

Cover the mould with a board, then towels or blankets as usual.

Cherry domino soap

Mmm, the cherry jam aroma fools me into thinking I'm stirring up something edible! When I dropped the dots onto the soap it reminded me of my mother's jam making and testing the jam for the setting stage.

LYE SOLUTION
168 g water • 63 g sodium hydroxide

SOAP OILS AND BUTTERS
200 g olive oil • 100 g cherry kernel oil • 100 g coconut oil
50 g shea butter

SOAP SCENT
12 g cherry fragrance oil

COLOUR
0.5 g autumn red mica

METHOD
Follow steps 1–7 of the cold process soap making steps (pages 37–8) until you have reached light trace. Add the cherry fragrance oil and stir again. Remove one tablespoon of the soap, add the autumn red mica to it and stir again.

Pour the uncoloured soap into the moulds and then drop four or five dots of red soap mixture onto the top of each bar. Insulate and leave for 24 hours.

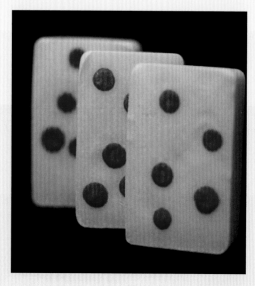

Cherry domino soap

MAKING SOAP USING THE HOT PROCESS METHOD

Whilst making soap using the hot process method can be a little tricky, the soap is ready to use as soon as it has hardened – this could be as little as two days – making it a popular choice for impatient soapers. It is a technique definitely worth perfecting if you don't want to wait the 4–6 week period that the cold process soap making usually takes.

The soap is hotter and harder when it goes into the mould so you do need to be prepared to work carefully and quickly. Your spoons and saucepan will be much easier to clean than they are from the cold process method, since this time the residue will be soapy rather than greasy.

There are a few more stages to making hot process soap than for the cold process method. I estimate that it will take about one and a half to two hours from weighing the ingredients to pouring your soap into the mould.

If you have a slow cooker (crock-pot) you don't have to stir your soap as often, since the heat is distributed more evenly throughout the soap mixture so reducing the risk of it burning.

The first part of your hot process soap making is to make up a batch of soap just as you would when making cold process soap. I have repeated the steps 1–7 here to help you.

Step 1
Get all your equipment, ingredients, safety wear and sundries ready. Line your mould if necessary and place to one side.

Step 2
Weigh the water required for the lye solution. Place the water jug to one side whilst you weigh the sodium hydroxide.

Step 3
Weigh the sodium hydroxide making sure that you adhere to all the safety instructions given in the section about handling sodium hydroxide (page 9).

Step 4
Carefully tip the sodium hydroxide into the water and stir until there is no gritty feeling at the bottom of the jug as this means that all the sodium hydroxide has dissolved.

Step 5
Weigh the oils, butters and waxes and transfer to a saucepan or slow cooker (crock-pot). Place on the heat until the solid oils, butters and waxes have melted. Do not include the essential or fragrance oils yet.

Step 6

Wearing safety goggles and gloves and paying careful attention to the safe handling of the lye, pour a very small amount of lye into the melted oils. If there is no reaction, such as the oils trying to fizz and react to the lye, carry on carefully pouring the lye into the melted oils.

Step 7

Stir the oils and lye together until they form a light trace. Whilst you can do this task by hand, you will find it much quicker to perform using a handheld stick blender. Blitz the soap mixture until it reaches trace. This will probably take about two or three minutes depending on the temperature of the oils, the ambient temperature and whether or not you have oils that may speed up or slow down reaching the trace stage.

Step 8

Hob method: place the traced soap in the saucepan back onto the hob and cook over a low heat, stirring every 10 minutes or so. If you have a lid for the saucepan, put it on the pan whilst the soap is cooking.
Slow cooker (crock-pot) method: place the lid on the slow cooker and leave the heat setting on medium or low.

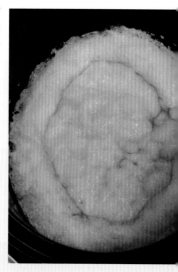

Step 9

Hob method: keep the heat low and do not allow the soap to overcook. Be aware that the soap mixture may trap air, causing it to rise up inside the saucepan. When stirring, do watch out for the soap mixture to puff up as it may volcano out of the saucepan. The soap will go through a phase referred to as 'apple sauce' since it looks very similar to puréed stewed apples.

Step 9: Hot process soap starting the gel phase

Slow cooker (crock-pot) method: keep an eye on the soap mixture and stir every 20 minutes.

When going in for the stir, place the spoon carefully in the saucepan in case it releases any trapped air. Always remember that this soap mixture is hot and caustic, so wear protective gloves at all times when stirring.

After 20 minutes or so you may notice that the edges of the mixture start to turn a little transparent. This is the soap gelling, which is what your cold process soap does itself when under towels and blankets. Stir the transparent parts of the soap back into the main soap mixture. Be sure to scrape down any soap that is resting on the inside walls of the saucepan or slow cooker (crock-pot). Keep stirring the soap thoroughly and regularly. When you are not stirring, prepare any other soap making ingredients you need, such as weighing out, your fragrance or essential oil. If you plan to colour your soap, you can add the colour at this stage and allow it to blend into the soap each time you stir it. Once the soap looks translucent and a little like a glossy Vaseline, the mixture is ready.

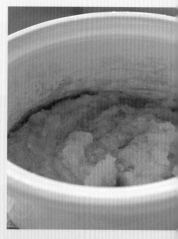

Step 9: Hot process soap reaching the apple sauce phase

Step 10

To make sure the soap mixture is ready, test a little to ensure that it has reached the correct consistency.

Take a little of the soap mixture (about half a teaspoon will do) and place it on a plate or saucer. Leave it to cool slightly and then touch it with your pointing finger, having removed your gloves first. Roll the soap mixture between finger and thumb; if it feels greasy or you can see an oily trail, the soap isn't ready yet so continue cooking and stirring for another 5–10 minutes.

If the soap mixture feels creamy, paste-like and rather like soap when rolled between finger and thumb then it is slightly more than done! Remove it from the heat. You'll soon get used to being able to spot the signs of your soap being ready – and the worst that can happen is that it becomes very thick and less easy to pour, and will not have a smooth surface.

Step 11

Add your fragrance and if you are planning to use any colour do so now, if you haven't already. Stir quickly and thoroughly to ensure that the colour and smell are evenly distributed into the soap mixture. Work quickly as the soap will start to harden up and it's best to get it into the mould whilst as fluid as possible. If it gets too hard or thick, add a little additional hot water to the soap mixture to make it slightly easier to handle and pour into the mould.

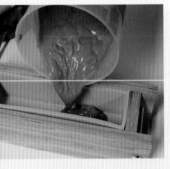

Step 12

Spoon, pour or dollop the soap mixture into your mould, pressing down to release any trapped air bubbles. When all the soap mixture is in, bang the mould down on the work surface to remove trapped air and to level off the top.

If the surface of the soap looks a little rugged, cover with a piece of polythene or cling film and smooth it out by stroking it.

Step 12: Pouring thick, hot process soap into the mould

Step 13

Leave the soap to harden in the mould. There is no need to insulate it during this time. Once the soap is hard enough to retain its own shape, remove from the mould. You can either leave the soap as a whole block or cut it into slices before leaving it at room temperature to harden up, which should only take a few days.

As soon as it is hard, the soap is ready for use.

SOAP RECIPES USING THE HOT PROCESS METHOD

When you have successfully made soap using the cold process method, do try to make soap using the hot process method. I remember the first time I made hot process soap – it is simple once you know what you're doing and unless I want to fiddle about doing some fancy colouring techniques, this is the method I prefer to use.

Smooth and luscious soap

The addition of tonka bean fragrance oil makes this soap smell fabulous. Tonka bean is mid-way between a chocolate and a vanilla smell and slowly changes the soap from ivory to beige. It is beautiful in looks and aroma.

LYE SOLUTION
168 g water • 60 g sodium hydroxide

SOAP OILS AND BUTTERS
200 g olive oil • 50 g coconut oil • 100 g castor oil
100 g sweet almond oil

SOAP SCENT
12 g tonka bean fragrance oil

METHOD
Follow the hot process soap making steps 1–11 (pages 47–9) and add the tonka bean fragrance oil. Stir well and quickly get your soap into the mould.

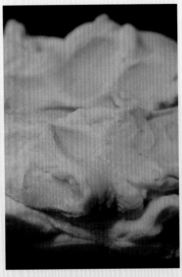

Smooth and luscious soap

Cooling, conditioning soap

The addition of peppermint essential oil makes this soap smell uplifting whilst having a cooling, tingling effect on the body. It is definitely an invigorating soap – perfect for your early morning ablutions. All the oils have linoleic and oleic acids, as does the cocoa butter, so this soap will be especially conditioning, leaving your skin feeling silky soft.

LYE SOLUTION
168 g water • 57 g sodium hydroxide

SOAP OILS AND BUTTERS
130 g olive oil • 80 g castor oil • 80 g avocado oil
80 g grapeseed oil • 80 g cocoa butter

SOAP SCENT
12 g peppermint essential oil

COLOUR
1 g blue ultramarine mixed with 10 g water

METHOD
Whilst waiting for the soap to cook, mix the ultramarine into 10 g water until the water has turned blue and the ultramarine has dissolved fully.

Follow steps 1–9 of the hot process soap making method (pages 47–9) and add the ultramarine blue liquid to the soap mixture whilst it cooks. Stir well.

Continue to step 11 and add the peppermint essential oil. Stir well and quickly get your soap into the mould.

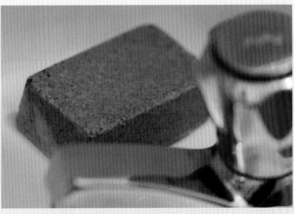

Cooling, conditioning soap

Herbal haven

The herbaceous aroma from the essential oils is stimulating, yet comforting. The oils chosen will create a big, richly lathered bar that leaves the skin feeling soft and moisturised, courtesy of the very generous dollop of shea butter.

LYE SOLUTION

168 g water • 61 g sodium hydroxide

SOAP OILS AND BUTTERS

50 g olive oil • 50 g palm oil • 100 g coconut oil
100 g castor oil • 150 g shea butter

COLOUR

2 g green clay mixed with 10 g olive oil

SOAP SCENT

6 g rosemary essential oil • 3 g lavender essential oil
2 g clary sage essential oil • 1 g basil essential oil

METHOD

Whilst waiting for the soap to cook, mix the green clay into 10 g olive oil (this is in addition to the olive oil used as part of the main soap recipe). Follow steps 1–9 of the hot process soap making method (pages 47–9) and add green oxide olive oil to the soap mixture whilst it cooks. Stir well.

Continue to step 11 and add the essential oils. Stir well and quickly get your soap into the mould.

Dirty mud and mango butter bar

I always smile at the irony of washing myself with a bar of soap containing mud. I've experimented with all sorts of aromas that I think are fitting with the mud and mango butter and this time I suggest that you use mostly mango, but with a dash of lime.

LYE SOLUTION
168 g water • 63 g sodium hydroxide

SOAP OILS AND BUTTERS
200 g olive oil • 100 g coconut oil • 90 g palm oil • 60 g mango butter

SOAP SCENT
9 g mango fragrance oil • 3 g lime essential oil

ADDITION
3 g Dead Sea mud (mixed with 10 g water)

METHOD
Whilst waiting for the soap to cook, mix the Dead Sea mud into 10 g water (this is in addition to the water used to make the lye). Follow steps 1–11 of the hot process soap making method (pages 47–9) and add the mango and lime blend. Stir well. Pour half your soap mixture into the mould and add the Dead Sea mud slurry to the remaining soap mixture in the saucepan. Stir well and pour a layer of mud soap on top of the uncoloured soap already in the mould.

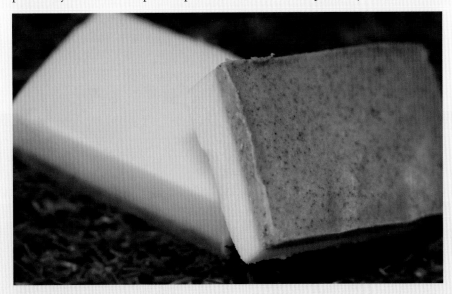

Dirty mud and mango butter bars

Peachy glow

There's lots of peach in this soap! I have selected peach kernel oil, peach fragrance oil and, if you can get them, crushed peach kernels to use as the mild exfoliating ingredient. If you can't get crushed peach kernels, substitute strawberry or poppy seeds.

LYE SOLUTION
168 g water • 63 g sodium hydroxide

SOAP OILS AND BUTTERS
100 g olive oil • 100 g coconut oil
200 g peach kernel oil • 50 g shea butter

SOAP SCENT
12 g peach fragrance oil

ADDITIONS
1 g crushed peach kernels • 20 g hot water

METHOD
Follow the hot process soap making steps 1–11 (pages 47–9) and add the peach fragrance oil. Working quickly, place half the soap in the mould. Add the crushed peach kernels and 20 g hot water to the remaining soap mixture and stir well. Pour the seeded soap into the mould on top of the non-seeded soap.

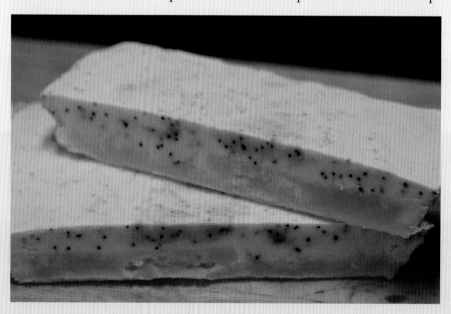

Peachy glow soap

Rosy hue soap

The cost of rose essential oil can make it prohibitive for use in soap unless you have an unlimited budget. Many floral fragrance oils are notorious for seizing (where the mixture suddenly goes very thick and becomes almost unmanageable due to the components of the fragrance oils – see page 25) and the rose we use is especially prone to this, so I have included rose geranium for its beautiful floral aroma. You'll be pleased to know that it behaves extremely well in soaps.

To team up with the beautiful aroma I have included some of my favourite oils. This is definitely one of my favourite soaps.

Lye solution
168 g water • 61 g sodium hydroxide

Soap oils and butters
100 g avocado oil • 80 g coconut oil • 160 g olive oil
50 g palm oil • 50 g shea butter • 10 g argan oil

Soap scent
12 g rose geranium essential oil (blended with another 10 g argan oil)

Colour
2 g pink mica (or infuse your olive oil with alkanet root for at least three weeks prior to making the soap. This will make the olive oil pink and eliminates the need for any additional colour).

Method
Follow the hot process soap making steps 1–11 (pages 47–8) and add the rose geranium oil blended with 10 g argan oil and the pink mica, if using.

Stir well and quickly get your soap into the mould. If you have time before the soap hardens up, blob a little pink soap on top and drag a teaspoon handle through it to create a swirled effect.

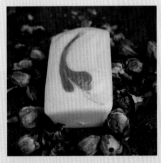

Rosy hue soap

Special effects using colour

As much as you may choose to make soap for its beautiful post-washing skin feel or lovely aroma, never underestimate the importance of its appearance either. We've had many a request to not only make soaps in the colour scheme of shower rooms and bathrooms, but also to create marbled, stripy and swirled soaps in various colours too. We even had a request to match a football kit! There are many colouring effects that you can beautify your soap with and if you are creative, here is your chance to make soap that really stands out.

Since many of the techniques require you to play around with coloured soap batter, you must make sure that you choose essential and fragrance oils that do not try to accelerate trace. One of the keys to successful colouring is to keep your soap very runny for as long as possible, so I would definitely only attempt the specialist colouring techniques with cold process soap. It's not advisable to discount the water or stick blend to anything other than a very runny trace: you need the maximum amount of time possible to pour the different colours.

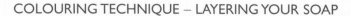

COLOURING TECHNIQUE – LAYERING YOUR SOAP

Layering your soap into two or three different stripes is one of the simplest colouring techniques. This technique can be carried out with a light to medium trace so it's a good one to adopt if your soap mixture starts to thicken up.

Split the runny soap batter into two or three portions and make each one a different colour.

Soap decorated using the feathering technique (page 59)

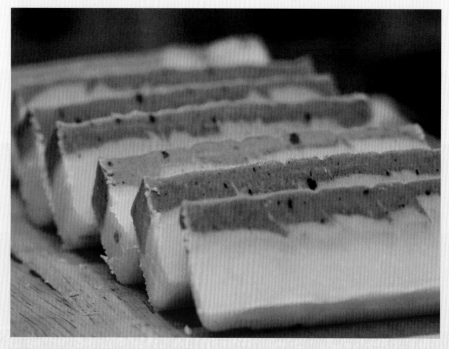

Cream, purple and pale pink

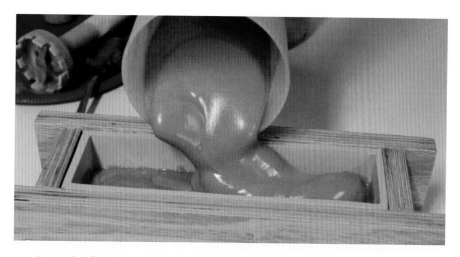

Pouring the second layer of soap

Pour the first layer and bang your mould down onto the work surface to remove any trapped air bubbles and to smooth out the surface of the soap. You need to pour the second layer as carefully as possible to avoid dislodging the first layer and blurring the line between the two. This may be easier if you pour the soap onto a spatula and allow it to drizzle off the spatula onto the first layer. Once you have poured the second layer, repeat with the third colour. Once all your layers are poured, cover and insulate your soap as usual (see page 38).

It is possible to have a perfectly straight edge where the two colours meet, but this will involve two stages. Make your soap as above but after you have poured the first coloured layer, cover with towels to insulate it and leave to rest for 24 hours. After 24 hours the soap will be hard, so pouring a new batch will mean that the second layer sits comfortably on top of the first without blending or merging the layers.

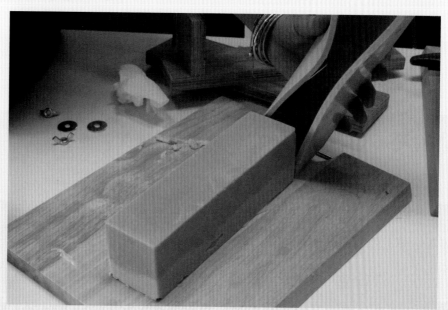

Green and beige layered soap

COLOURING TECHNIQUE – CHUNKING YOUR SOAP

Chunking is another easy colouring technique and a very useful method of using up odd bits of coloured soap! If you don't have any odd bits of soap to hand, the chunking technique will need to be carried out over a few days.

If you don't have odd bits of soap, make up a small, 200 g block of scented, highly coloured soap. Cover, insulate and leave it for 24 hours. After 24 hours remove from the mould and cut into small, 1 cm squares or chunks and set to one side. If you do have approximately 200 g of odd bits of soap, cut these into 1 cm chunks and set to one side.

You will need a mould that can hold at least 800 g of soap. Make up a 600g batch of soap, bring it to light trace and add the fragrance. Stir the soap mixture well. If you plan to colour this outer layer, choose a shade that is significantly different from the colour of the chunks so they contrast beautifully.

Place the chunks in your soap batter and give a quick stir to make sure they are evenly distributed throughout the mixture. Pour into your mould and bang the mould onto the work surface to dislodge any bubbles. Cover and insulate as usual before cutting into slices once it is ready.

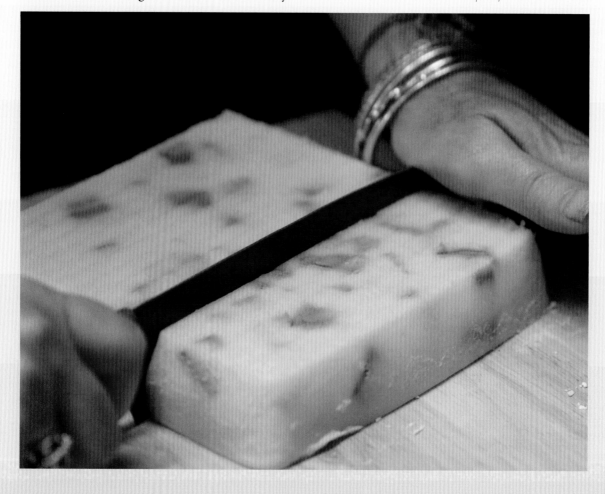

Cutting the chunked soap loaf

COLOURING TECHNIQUE – FEATHERING YOUR SOAP

The feathering technique can be applied to the top of your soap to make bars look a little like a rather tasty cream slice. Exactly the same technique is used by patissiers.

This technique will require that your soap batter is on the runny side, so bring to a very light trace only. Add the fragrance and stir well. Remove 30–60 g of the soap base and place in a jug. Add the colouring to the mixture in the jug and stir well (if it starts to thicken up, add a little hot water to make it runny again).

Remove another 30–60 g uncoloured soap and place in a different jug. Add a different colour to this jug and mix.

Pour the larger batch of scented soap into your mould and bang the mould onto the work surface to smooth the top and remove any air bubbles.

Pour the first coloured soap in the jug onto the soap in the mould by drizzling thin stripes of soap lengthways across the top of the soap. If you can pour from a height it will help the coloured soap to sink into the main soap a little rather than just sit on top.

Repeat using the second colour to create alternate stripes.

When you have thin stripes of soap on top of the main soap, stop pouring and set any remaining coloured soap aside as this isn't needed now. You can pour it into a different mould to make a solid colour soap.

Insert the tip of a metal skewer, wooden chopstick or other thin utensil into the edge of the soap about 2 cm along the first stripe that you poured. Carefully but steadily pull the skewer across the stripes to the other edge of the soap (the coloured stripes should flow towards the pull and create a feathered look). Remove the skewer and give it a wipe. Repeat the pulling across the stripes but

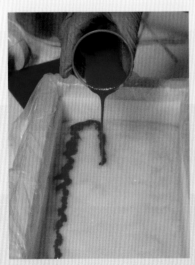

The first coloured stripe for the feathering technique

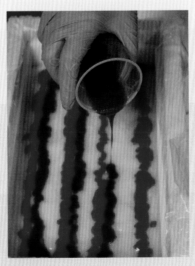

The second coloured stripe for the feathering technique

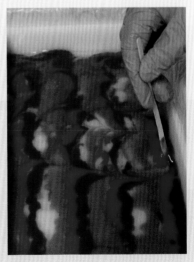

Pulling the stripes to create the feathered effect

this time start at the other side of the soap and work in the opposite direction.

Repeat the pulling of the skewer from side to side until the whole of the top of your soap has a feathered pattern across it.

Once you've mastered the art of feathering, experiment by feathering three or more different coloured stripes. You can create wonderful spider's web patterns by pouring soap into thin circles and then feathering by dragging your skewer or cocktail stick from the middle outwards.

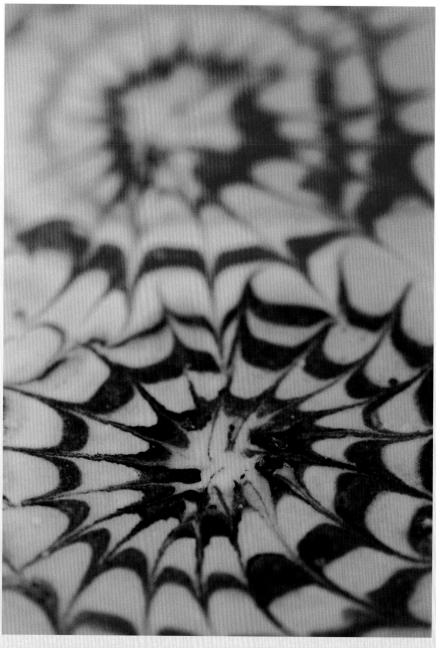

Circles instead of stripes are equally effective

COLOURING TECHNIQUE – SWIRLING YOUR SOAP

An alternative to feathering the surface of your soap is to swirl the surface instead. Repeat the exercise for feathering, but instead of pulling your skewer from side to side, draw small circles in the stripes and drag the coloured stripes in different directions. Be careful not to drag too many times in case the colours start to merge into one and you lose the delicate patterns.

Swirled soap can look breathtakingly beautiful, especially if the swirls continue into the soap rather than just sit on the top. There are various methods of achieving this and, with experience, soap makers tend to develop their own preferred method.

When swirling the colours in your soap, be prepared for a few surprises as swirling doesn't always go to plan. Please don't worry if it doesn't work out exactly as you intended – the results will still be beautiful.

Golden swirled soap

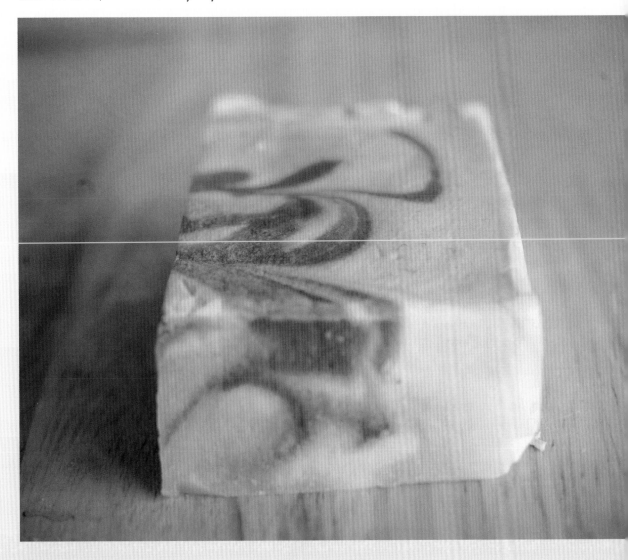

In-pot swirl

The 'in-pot' swirl is probably the easiest method of swirling. In the example here I shall describe how to do an in-pot swirl with three different coloured portions of soap and one uncoloured portion, but you can swirl with as many different colours as you wish.

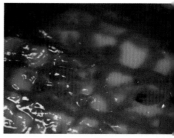

Purple and green swirled in the saucepan

If your mould needs lining, prepare it and place to one side. Now prepare your colours. Place the first colour that you have chosen to use in a small container. If you are using a powdered colour, I recommend that you add a little water or oil to it so that it becomes a liquid colour.

Repeat placing your two other liquid colours in different small containers.

Bring your soap to a very light trace and add the fragrances (make sure you choose fragrances that won't accelerate trace, see page 25). Stir the soap mixture well.

When you have made sure that the fragrance or essential oils are thoroughly incorporated into the soap mixture, pour about a quarter of it into the small container containing the colour and stir well.

Repeat until you have three small containers of different coloured soap and a quarter of the soap mixture uncoloured and still in the saucepan. You will need to work fairly quickly before the soap tries to thicken up.

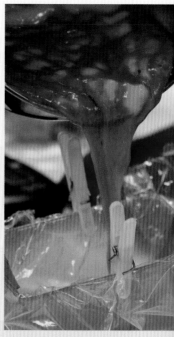

Take the small container holding the first colour and drizzle the colour back into the saucepan. Pour from a height as this will help the coloured soap to fall into the uncoloured soap mixture rather than just sit on the surface. Drizzle thin stripes of soap in lines back and forth over the uncoloured soap in the saucepan.

When you have used up the first coloured soap, repeat the exercise by pouring the coloured soap in the second small container back into the saucepan. Drizzle soap in stripes across the other soaps in the pan.

Repeat with the third small container until all your soap is back in the saucepan. ***Do not stir the soap in the saucepan at any stage of the colouring process.***

Now carefully pour the stripy coloured soap in the saucepan into the mould. Some of the soap colours will merge together whilst others will stay as stripes – no matter how it ends up, it will look amazing!

Cover and insulate for 24 hours as usual before cutting into stripes and admiring your work.

Pouring the swirled colours

In-mould swirl

The 'in-mould' swirl is similar to the in-pot swirl but this time all the pouring and swirling is done in the mould and not the saucepan. As with the in-pot swirl, prepare two or three coloured portions of soap, leaving one portion uncoloured. Again you can swirl with as many different colours as you wish.

If your mould needs lining, prepare it and place to one side. Prepare your colours in the small containers so that they are ready to be stirred into the portioned-off soap mixture.

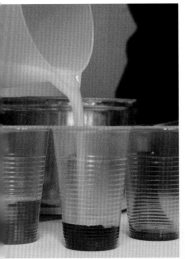

Preparing the different coloured soap mixtures

Bring your soap to a very, very light trace and add the fragrance. Pour the first portion of soap to be coloured into a little container and blend in the colour so that is it evenly distributed throughout.

Repeat until you have different coloured soap in little containers ready to pour into the mould. Pour a drizzle of the first coloured soap into your mould, making sure that you have a stripe running from one end of the mould to the other. The mixture should remain in stripes and not cover the entire base.

Take the jug with the second colour and pour another drizzle of soap running next to the first soap that you poured.

Repeat using the third coloured soap and then the uncoloured soap. Once you have drizzled all four quarters of soap (three coloured and one uncoloured), repeat the exercise again, pouring a drizzle of the first colour on top of the soap already in the mould.

Repeat with all the colours time and again until you have no soap mixture left.

Cover and insulate for 24 hours as usual before cutting the block of soap into attractive individual slices.

Coat-hanger swirl

The technique called the coat-hanger swirl is an extension of the in-mould swirl. A wire coat hanger is all that is needed as your swirling tool. You will be using one of the triangular corners and inserting it temporarily into your mould, so make sure it actually fits into the mould before you start to pour the soap. If necessary, bend or squash it to make it thinner.

Using the in-pot swirl instructions (page 62), pour layers of coloured soap into the mould. Once all the soap is inside, carefully insert the triangular corner of the coat hanger into the soap at one end of the mould, so that it is touching the bottom of the mould, being careful not to dislodge the liner if you are using one.

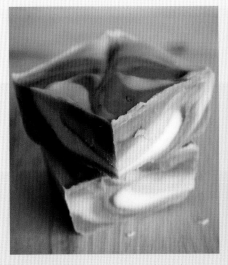

Swirls and colours running throughout the soap

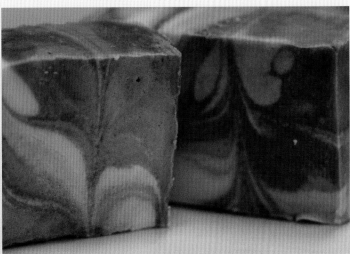

Beautifully swirled soap made using the coat-hanger swirl method

Slowly bring the coat hanger up towards the surface of the soap, moving it a few centimetres along the soap as you lift it. When you have almost reached the top of the soap, move the coat hanger down into the soap again, moving a couple of centimetres along the soap as you push it back down. When you reach the bottom of the soap again your coat hanger should be further along the soap, having moved in a wave throughout the full height of the soap.

Repeat the wave movement from top to bottom throughout the soap until you reach the other end of the mould. Carefully remove the coat hanger from the soap and wipe it clean.

Cover and insulate your soap for 24 hours before cutting it into slices.

Note: this technique can also be carried out using a chopstick or long teaspoon handle instead of a coat hanger although I think the final effect of having used the coat hanger is more visually pleasing.

Faux funnel swirl

The faux funnel swirl is so called because it is based on a method that was originally carried out by pouring your soap into a funnel carefully placed above the mould. The new method has done away with using a funnel. It gives a similar effect, but is quicker and less messy. Split your very, very lightly traced fragranced soap batch into three or four smaller batches and add colour to each one (you can leave one portion uncoloured if you wish). It is important that your soap is runny and easy to pour, so work quickly. If it starts to thicken up, continuing with the faux funnel swirl will not be easy and you may even have to start again.

Pour about two tablespoons of your first colour into the middle of the mould. It will sit there creating a little puddle of soap.

Now take your second colour and pour approximately two tablespoons of this directly into the middle of the other coloured soap puddle. As you pour, it will displace the original soap puddle, moving it out towards the edge of the mould.

Take your third colour and pour a similar small amount directly into the centre

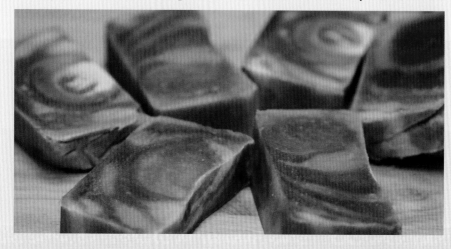

Soaps made using the faux funnel swirl technique

of the second colour that you poured, allowing the soap to be displaced as before.

Continue pouring a little of each colour directly into the centre of the previously poured puddle, allowing the soap to gradually fill up the mould. Repeat until you have no soap mixture left.

Cover and insulate for 24 hours before cutting into amazingly impressive slices.

Randomly poured faux funnel swirls

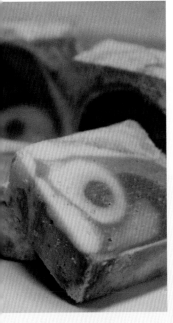

Faux funnel swirl II

A slight variation on the faux funnel swirl but just as easy.

Prepare your very, very lightly traced fragranced soap, split into portions and colour each one. This time, rather than pouring a puddle of soap into the centre of the mould, pour a small puddle at one end of the mould and another identically coloured puddle at the other end.

You will now have two coloured puddles in your soap mould. Take the second colour and pour another little puddle of this coloured soap into each of the puddles already placed in the mould. Repeat until you have poured a couple of puddles of each of the coloured soap mixture.

Take your first coloured soap and pour another two puddles at different locations in your soap mould and build on these puddles as before until you have poured two layers of coloured puddles.

Again, take your first coloured soap and pour another two puddles elsewhere in the soap mould. By now your soap will be looking a little psychedelic with swirls and puddles all over the place (but hopefully only in the mould!). Continue pouring and building up random soap puddles until the mixture has been used up.

Cover and insulate the soap for 24 hours before cutting into kaleidoscopic-looking slices.

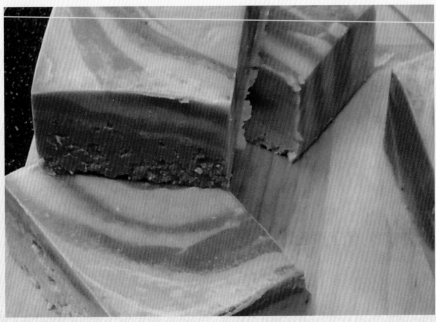

Swirls in the strawberry soap

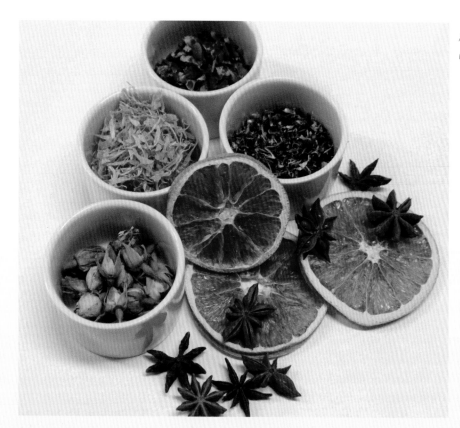

A selection of botanicals to use in traditional soap

Using botanicals, fruit and vegetables in your soap

Fresh and dried botanicals, fruit and vegetables can all be used in your cold process soaps in a number of different ways.

BOTANICAL DECORATIONS IN SOAP

The most obvious method is to include dried petals or leaves in your soap or as decorations scattered on top of the soap just before you place it under blankets and towels for 24 hours. Whilst these can look hugely attractive initially, most botanicals will brown overtime and make the soap look less appealing.

Rosebuds and cloves inserted into soap can look very pretty and may enhance the aroma of soap. But these soaps aren't practical to use as the rosebuds and cloves will need to be removed before use, leaving little brown marks in the soap at the insertion point. I have found that you can help reduce the browning by pouring a thin layer of melted cocoa butter onto the surface of the soap when you remove it from its blankets after the first 24 hours.

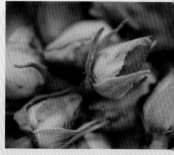

Let the cocoa butter set softly and insert the rosebuds or other plant material into the cocoa butter. Leave for a few hours so that the cocoa butter sets hard before slicing the soap.

Rosebuds can look very pretty, but aren't always practical

*Infusing nettles and
alkanet root*

Poppy seeds, rosehips, cranberry seeds, raspberry seeds, oats (as in oatmeal – yes, porridge oats!) can all be used in or on your soaps too. Poppy seeds keep their grey colouring whilst porridge oats will retain their beige to brown colour. The other seeds mentioned will turn from light brown to a darker shade of brown.

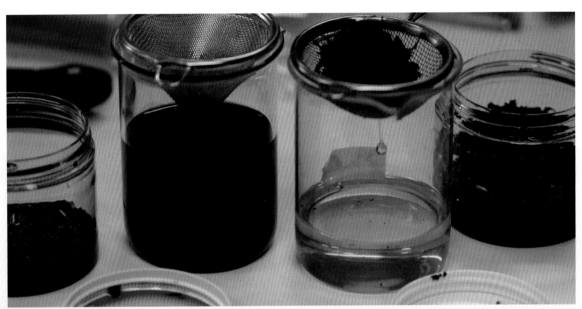

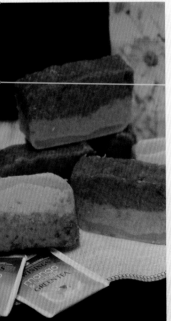

BOTANICAL INFUSIONS IN SOAP

Another method of including the properties of the botanicals such as dried rose petals, nettles, calendula (marigold) petals, rosemary, mint and other herbs in your soap is to infuse the plant material in olive oil and store in a lidded bottle or jar for a few weeks at room temperature.

Filter out the plant material and use the olive oil as part of your soap base. It is unlikely that much, if any, aroma from the plant material will be included in your soap, but some of its properties will have been transferred into the oil and therefore into your soap.

FRUIT AND HERBAL TEAS IN SOAP

Teas such as green tea, rosehip, rooibos, fruit, chamomile and lemongrass can also be used in your soaps. Their natural properties will also be transferred to the soap. Remove the tea leaves from the tea bags and scatter tea leaves into or onto your soap, or use the cold tea as part of your lye solution.

FRUIT AND VEGETABLE PURÉES

*Layered soap made with
mango and lychee green
tea bags*

An interesting and appealing method of including botanicals, fruits and vegetables in your soap is to purée the plant material with a little water and include as part of the soap. Please note that this is more likely to be successful with cold process or no-heat soaps.

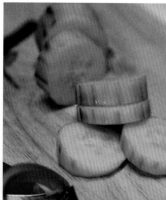

Peeled and chopped cucumber, ready to be puréed

Fruit and vegetables that you might consider using include strawberries, figs, mangos, avocados, cucumber, carrots, bananas, pumpkin, sweet potatoes, lettuce, peaches, oranges, kiwi fruits … but the list is not limited to these fruit and vegetables only. Have fun experimenting!

Do note that any fruit with pips, such as strawberries and kiwi fruit, will make an exfoliating bar. You may wish to sieve the purée to remove the pips before use.

Dried fruit can be used as well. For the best results, soak in water overnight to rehydrate and plump the fruit up. Drain the water off and use it as your lye water.

I cannot vouch for the final colour of the soap – and many of the fruit and vegetables mentioned above will turn your soap brown. We always used to colour our strawberry soap red – brown strawberry soap just doesn't look tempting!

There is a general myth that putting herbs, vegetables and fruit into your soap will require a preservative. This is not true as the saponification process will kill off any 'nasties' that you may have inadvertently introduced with these additions. It is good practice, however to wash any fresh fruit (or similar) in a baby sterilising solution such as Milton prior to use (if you plan to peel it, washing isn't strictly necessary).

CALCULATING HOW MUCH FRUIT AND VEGETABLES TO USE IN YOUR SOAP

Before starting your fruit or vegetable soap making session you will need to work out how much purée to add. My rule of thumb is to use between 5 and 10 per cent of the total weight of the base soap ingredients, excluding the weight of the sodium hydroxide. So if your oils, butters, waxes and water come to a weight of 600 g, you would need between 30 and 60 g of purée. This calculation is performed by taking the total weight of your soap and dividing it by 100 to get 1 per cent. Multiply the value of 1 per cent by 5 to get the minimum amount of purée weight and by 10 to get the maximum amount of purée weight.

600/100 = 6 (so 6 g is the value of 1 per cent)
6 x 5 = 30 (so 30 g is the minimum amount of purée to use)
6 x 10 = 60 (so 60 g is the maximum amount of purée to use)

PREPARING YOUR FRUIT PURÉE

Wash the fruit in a sterilising solution unless you plan to peel it, in which case washing isn't necessary. Drain to remove any excess moisture. Place the fruit in a liquidiser and add an equal amount of water, taken from the water you plan to use for the lye.

Wash the vegetables in a sterilising solution or peel them instead. If the fruit or vegetables are too hard to purée, cook them until they are soft enough. Now make a purée by putting them into a liquidiser with an equal weight of water removed from the water you have set aside to make the lye with. Pulverise the fruit and the water together until you have a smooth purée, making sure that there are no lumps of unpuréed fruit left. Strain through a sieve to remove any pips unless you intend to make an exfoliating bar, in which case keep the pips in.

PREPARING YOUR VEGETABLE PURÉE

Wash the vegetables in a sterilising solution or peel them instead. If they are too hard or fibrous to purée when raw, boil until they are soft enough. Now make a purée by putting them into a liquidiser with an equal weight of water taken from the water you have set aside to make the lye with. Pulverise until you have a smooth purée with no trace of any lumps. If you wish to use the vegetables raw (the colour will be more intense), grate into very thin shreds and place in a liquidiser with an equal amount of water reserved to make the lye. Pulverise until you have a smooth liquid with no traces of unpuréed shredded vegetables.

It is very important to note that your lye solution will be made with less water than usual since the purée contains some of the water you would normally include in the lye and the fruit and vegetables themselves contain a natural element of water.

Soaps made with botanicals, fruit and vegetable purées will have a shelf life of at least 18 months and do not require a preservative.

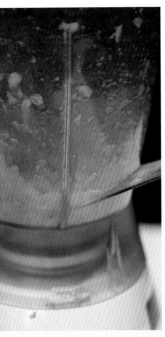

Chopped cucumber puréed in the liquidiser

FRUIT AND VEGETABLE SOAP RECIPES

In the recipes that follow I have included the purées using 5 per cent of the total weight of the soap ingredients. This gives sufficient interest and appeal, but it won't add a natural fruity or vegetable aroma to the soaps. I have picked fragrance or essential oils that blend nicely with the purées, but of course you can substitute these for your own preferred aroma blends.

Refer to the detailed cold process soap making instructions in the soap making methods section (page 37–8) and carry out steps 1–6 but include making the purée as well. I have included an overview of the steps for each recipe to help you.

USING DRIED FRUIT IN SOAPS

Whilst the recipes use fresh fruit and vegetables, you can replace the fresh fruit with dried fruit. Soak in water for at least six hours or, better still, overnight. Drain the fruit and pulverise with a little water in a liquidiser to create a manageable purée. Continue making your soap as you would if you were using fresh fruit. If you wish, you can use the discarded soaking water as the water in your lye solution.

Peachy perfection

Even more peaches in this soap than Peachy glow (page 54)! Peach kernel oil, peach fragrance and pure peach purée …

PEACH PURÉE
30 g peach flesh, chopped into small pieces • 30 g water

LYE SOLUTION
138 g water • 63 g sodium hydroxide

SOAP OILS AND BUTTERS
100 g olive oil • 100 g coconut oil • 200 g peach kernel oil
50 g shea butter

SOAP SCENT
12 g peach fragrance oil

METHOD
Line your mould if necessary and place it to one side.

Place your peach pieces and 30 g water in a liquidiser and pulverise until you have a smooth purée. Set aside.

Wearing safety equipment (page 10), make up your lye solution using 138 g water and 63 g sodium hydroxide. Set aside somewhere safely out of reach of children and pets.

Weigh the oils and shea butter and place in a saucepan. Set the pan on a low heat until the butter has melted.

Wearing safety goggles and gloves and paying careful attention to the safe handling of the lye (page 9), pour the lye into the melted butter and oils mixture.

Stir briefly with a spoon to mix the oils and lye together.

Add the peach purée and blitz with a handheld stick blender until you have reached light trace and you can see a line of soap mixture sitting on the surface when you drizzle the soap mixture onto the soap in the saucepan.

Add the peach fragrance oil and stir again.

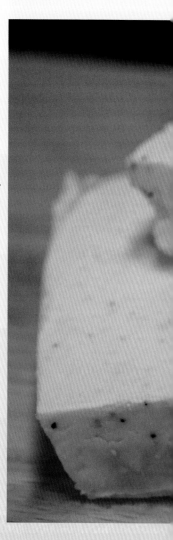

Pour the soap mixture into your prepared mould. Cover the mould with a lid, a chopping board or piece of cardboard to prevent the towels from falling into the soap.

Place a layer of old towels over the covered mould and leave for 24 hours before removing the soap from the mould.

Peachy perfection soap

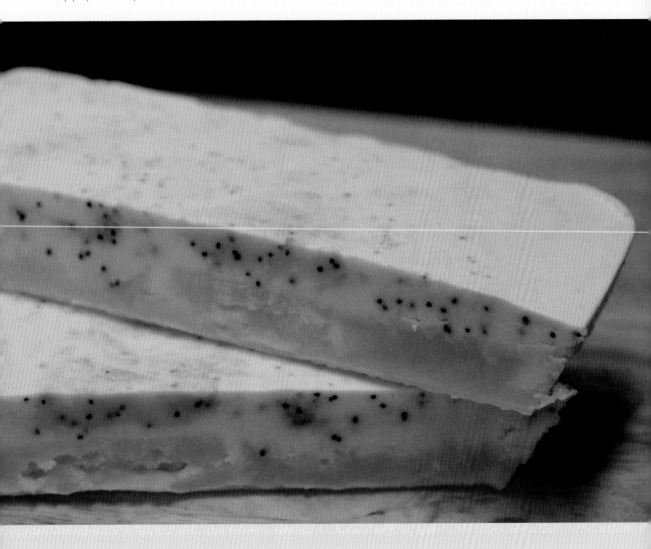

Cool as a cucumber

Cucumber tends to make the lye go slightly brown, so I have added a little liquid green CP soap colouring to make it look more authentic. I also suggest that you include a small amount of cucumber peel cut into tiny pieces to give a speckled effect.

Since cucumber has a high natural water content, I haven't added as much water to the purée.

CUCUMBER PURÉE
30 g cucumber, chopped into small pieces
5 g cucumber peel, cut into thin slivers
20 g water

LYE SOLUTION
148 g water • 65 g sodium hydroxide

SOAP OILS
200 g olive oil • 150 g coconut oil • 100 g palm oil

COLOUR
1 teaspoon green CP soap colour

SOAP SCENT
12 g cucumber fragrance oil

METHOD
Line your mould if necessary and place to one side.

Place the cucumber pieces (but not the extra peel) and 20 g water in a liquidiser; pulverise until you have a smooth purée. Add the cucumber peel slivers and set the cucumber purée aside.

Wearing safety equipment (page 10), make up the lye solution using 148 g water and 65 g sodium hydroxide. Set aside somewhere out of reach of children and pets. Weigh the oils and put them into a saucepan, then set the pan on a low heat until everything has melted.

Wearing safety goggles and gloves and paying careful attention to the safe handling of the lye (page 9), pour the lye into the melted oils mixture.

Stir briefly with a spoon to mix the oils and lye together.

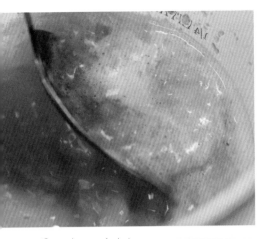

Add the cucumber purée and the green CP soap colour. Blitz with a handheld stick blender until you have reached light trace. Add the pieces of cucumber peel and stir well.

Add the cucumber fragrance oil and stir again.

Pour the soap mixture into your prepared mould. Cover the mould with a lid, chopping board or a piece of cardboard to prevent the towels from falling into the soap.

Cover the covered mould with a layer of old towels and leave for 24 hours before removing the soap from the mould.

Cucumber purée being mixed into the lye solution

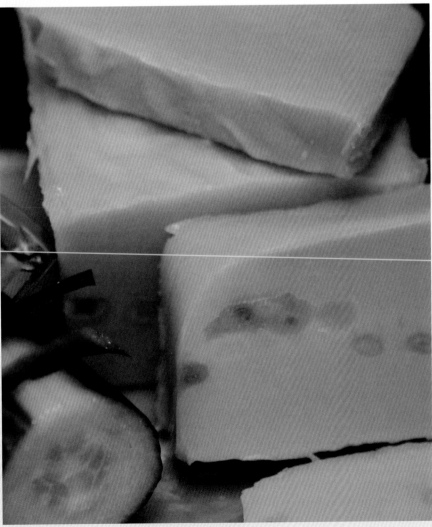

Cool as a cucumber soap

Strawberry smoothie

The natural colour of the strawberry soap is a milky coffee shade so you will definitely want to add red to give it more strawberry appeal. I have chosen to swirl this soap and, if you look closely, you will see I have left in a few strawberry seeds.

STRAWBERRY PURÉE
30 g strawberries, husk and stalks removed • 30 g water

LYE SOLUTION
138 g water • 61 g sodium hydroxide

SOAP OILS AND BUTTERS
200 g olive oil • 150 g coconut oil • 50 g beeswax • 50 g shea butter

COLOUR
2 teapoons red CP soap colour

SOAP SCENT
12 g strawberry fragrance oil

METHOD
Line your mould if necessary and place to one side.

Place the strawberries and 30 g water into a liquidiser; pulverise until you have a smooth purée. Pass through a sieve to remove the seeds; if you prefer, you may keep some seeds for a mildly exfoliating soap.

Wearing safety equipment (page 10), make up your lye solution using 138 g water and 61 g sodium hydroxide. Set aside somewhere out of reach of children and pets.

Weigh the oils and shea butter and put them into a saucepan. Set the pan on a low heat until everything has melted.

Wearing safety goggles and gloves and paying careful attention to the safe handling of the lye (page 9), pour the lye into the mixture of melted butter and oils.

Stir briefly with a spoon to mix the oils and lye together.

Add the strawberry purée. Blitz with a handheld stick blender until you have reached light trace.

Add the strawberry fragrance oil and stir again. Remove a little of the soap mixture and add the red CP soap colour to this.

Pour the uncoloured soap mixture into your prepared mould and swirl in the red mixture. Cover the mould with a lid, chopping board or a piece of cardboard to prevent the towels from falling into the soap.

Cover the covered mould with a layer of old towels and leave for 24 hours before removing the soap from the mould.

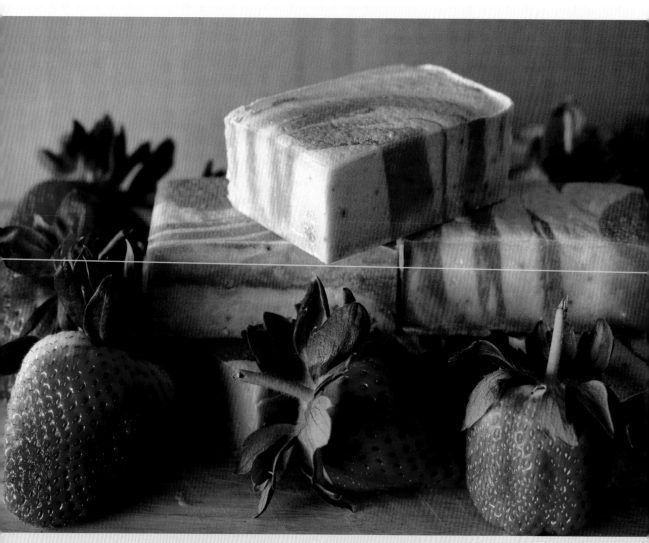

Strawberry smoothie soap

Sweet potato mash soap

We love sweet potato so keeping some aside to use in soap is the greatest challenge here! The beautiful orange colour from the vegetable transfers into the soap, turning it a glorious soft amber. Unrefined palm oil (available at large supermarkets) further enhances the natural orange colour.

Choosing a fragrance that keeps the sweet potato theme going was difficult. You can get parsnip essential oil but it is horribly expensive (it smells lovely in case you were wondering). Next time you are cooking parsnips, break a raw parsnip in half and take a big sniff. Inhale the aroma – it's wonderful!

In the end I went for essential oils of sweet orange and carrot seed, which blend well and sustain the root vegetable, orange and sweet potato fragrances.

Sweet potato purée
30 g peeled sweet potato, chopped into small pieces (boil the sweet potato until it is just turning soft)
20 g water

Lye solution
148 g water • 61 g sodium hydroxide

Soap oils and butters
250 g olive oil • 50 g coconut oil • 100 g unrefined palm oil
50 g cocoa butter

Soap scent
9 g sweet orange essential oil • 3 g carrot seed essential oil

Method
Line your mould if necessary and place to one side.

Place the sweet potato pieces and 20 g water into a liquidiser; pulverise until you have a smooth purée.

Wearing safety equipment (page 10), make up your lye solution using 148 g water and 61 g sodium hydroxide. Set aside somewhere out of reach of children and pets.

Weigh the oils and cocoa butter and put them into a saucepan. Set the pan on a low heat until everything has melted.

Wearing safety goggles and gloves and paying careful attention to the safe handling of the lye (page 9), pour the lye into the mixture of melted butter and oils.

Stir briefly with a spoon to mix the oils and lye together.

Add the sweet potato purée and blitz with a handheld stick blender until you have reached light trace and you can see a line of soap mixture sitting on the surface when you drizzle the soap mixture onto the soap in the saucepan.

Add the sweet orange and carrot seed essential oils and stir again.

Pour the soap mixture into your prepared mould.

Cover the mould with a lid, chopping board or a piece of cardboard to prevent the towels from falling into the soap. Now cover the covered mould with a layer of old towels and leave for 24 hours before removing the soap from the mould.

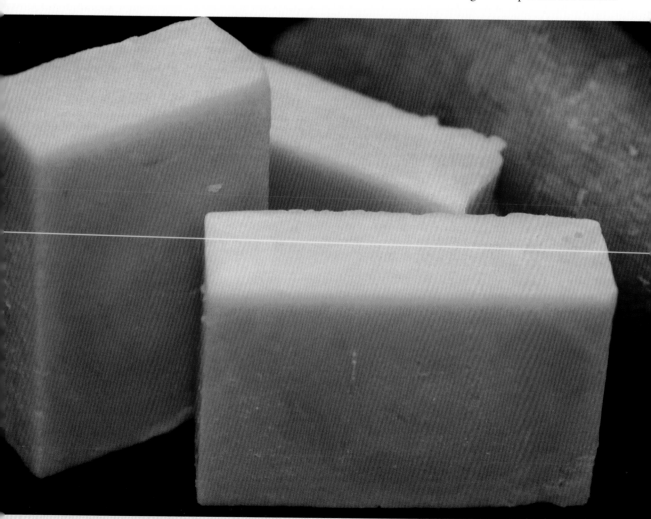

Sweet potato mash soap

Banana and mango butter bars

BANANA PURÉE
30 g banana, mashed • 30 g water

LYE SOLUTION
138 g water • 63 g sodium hydroxide

SOAP OILS AND BUTTERS
100 g coconut oil • 150 g olive oil • 100 g sweet almond oil
100 g mango butter

SOAP SCENT
6 g mango fragrance oil • 6 g banana fragrance oil

COLOUR
0.5g autumn red mica

METHOD
Line your mould if necessary and place to one side.

Place your mashed banana and 30 g water into a liquidiser; pulverise until you have a smooth purée.

Wearing safety equipment (page 10), make up your lye solution using 138 g water and 63 g sodium hydroxide. Set aside somewhere out of reach of children and pets.

Weigh the oils and mango butter and put them into a saucepan. Place the pan over a low heat until everything has melted.

Wearing safety goggles and gloves and paying careful attention to the safe handling of the lye (page 9), pour the lye into the mixture of melted butter and oils.

Stir briefly with a spoon to mix the oils and lye together.

Add the banana purée and blitz with a handheld stick blender until you have reached light trace.

Add the mango and banana fragrance oils and stir again.

Remove one third of the soap mixture and add the mica to this portion; stir well.

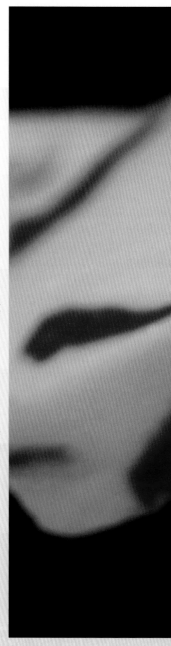

Pour a little of the uncoloured soap mixture into your prepared mould. Add a little of the red mica portion. Repeat, adding patches of uncoloured then red mica soap until you have used up all the soap mixture.

Cover the mould with a lid, chopping board or a piece of cardboard to prevent the towels from falling into the soap. Now cover the covered mould with a layer of old towels and leave for 24 hours before removing the soap from the mould.

Banana and mango butter bars

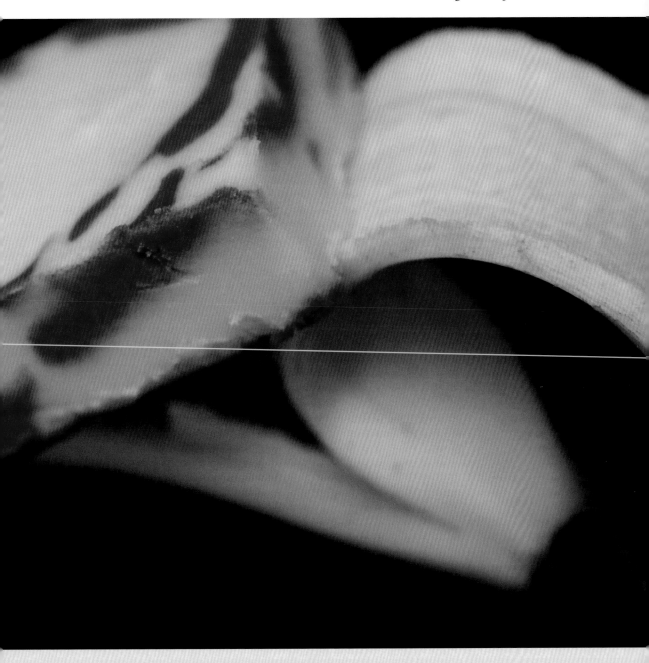

Carrot and orange bar

I can't recall how many times I've accidentally called this carrot and orange *soup* rather than soap! I've used dried orange slices to decorate the soap, with both carrot tissue oil and grated carrots to boost the carrot content.

CARROT PURÉE
30 g grated carrot • 30 g water

LYE SOLUTION
138 g water • 62 g sodium hydroxide

SOAP OILS
150 g olive oil • 100 g coconut oil • 50 g palm oil • 100 g rice bran oil
50 g carrot tissue oil

SOAP SCENT
12 g orange essential oil

ADDITION
Dried orange slices

METHOD
Line your mould if necessary and place to one side.

Place 30 g grated carrot with 30 g water into a liquidiser; pulverise until you have a smooth pulp.

Wearing safety equipment (page 10), make up your lye solution using 138 g water and 62 g sodium hydroxide. Set aside somewhere out of reach of children and pets.

Weigh the oils and put them into a saucepan. Set the pan over a low heat until everything has melted.

Wearing safety goggles and gloves and paying careful attention to the safe handling of the lye (page 9), pour the lye into the melted oils mixture.

Stir briefly with a spoon to mix the oils and lye together.

Add the carrot purée and blitz with a handheld stick blender until you have reached a light trace.

Add the orange essential oil and mix well.

Pour the soap mixture into the prepared mould and smooth down the surface. Carefully place slices of dried orange on top.

Cover the mould with a lid, chopping board or a piece of cardboard to prevent the towels from falling into the soap. Now cover the covered mould with a layer of old towels and leave for 24 hours before removing the soap from the mould.

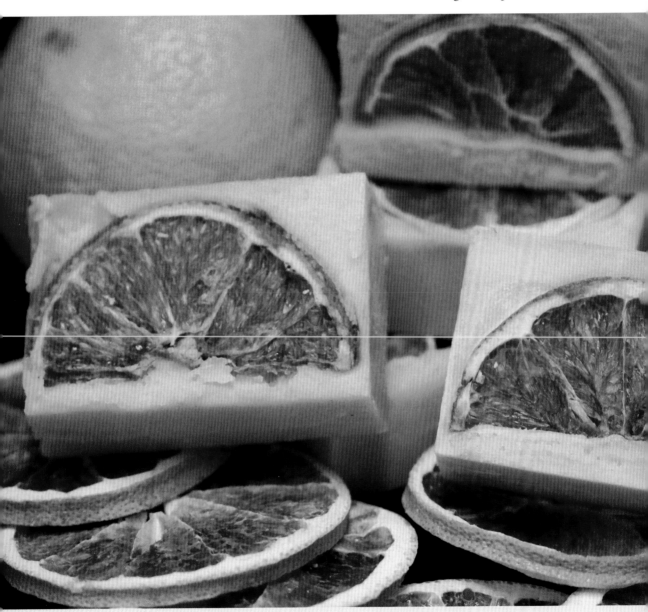

Carrot and orange bars

Pass the salad

I grow lettuces but I can't eat them as quickly as I grow them, so this is a fabulous summer soap that helps me use up the glut from the garden. You might consider adding cucumber or tomato purée too – or both – but I've only included the lettuce purée in this particular recipe.

LETTUCE PURÉE
30 g shredded lettuce • 30 g water

LYE SOLUTION
138 g water • 63 g sodium hydroxide

SOAP OILS
220 g olive oil • 100 g coconut oil • 80 g palm oil • 50 g sesame seed oil

COLOUR
$^{1}/_{2}$ teaspoon green CP soap colour

SOAP SCENT
6 g cucumber fragrance oil • 6 g lemon verbena essential oil

METHOD
Line your mould if necessary and place to one side.

Place the shredded lettuce with 30 g water in a liquidiser; pulverise until you have a smooth purée.

Wearing safety equipment (page 10), make up your lye solution using 138 g water and 63 g sodium hydroxide. Set aside somewhere out of reach of children and pets.

Weigh the oils and put them into a saucepan (there is no need to heat these oils).

Wearing safety goggles and gloves and paying careful attention to the safe handling of the lye (page 9), pour the lye into the oils mixture.

Stir briefly with a spoon to mix the oils and lye together. Add the green CP soap colouring.

Add the lettuce purée and blitz with a handheld stick blender until you have reached a light trace.

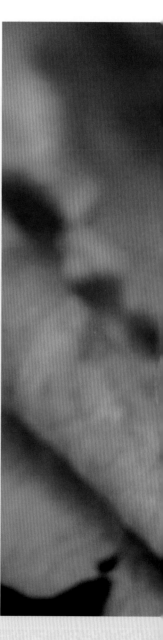

Add the cucumber fragrance oil and lemon verbena essential oil to the soap mixture and stir well.

Pour the soap mixture into your prepared mould.

Cover the mould with a lid, chopping board or a piece of cardboard to prevent the towels from falling into the soap. Now cover the covered mould with a layer of old towels and leave for 24 hours before removing the soap from the mould.

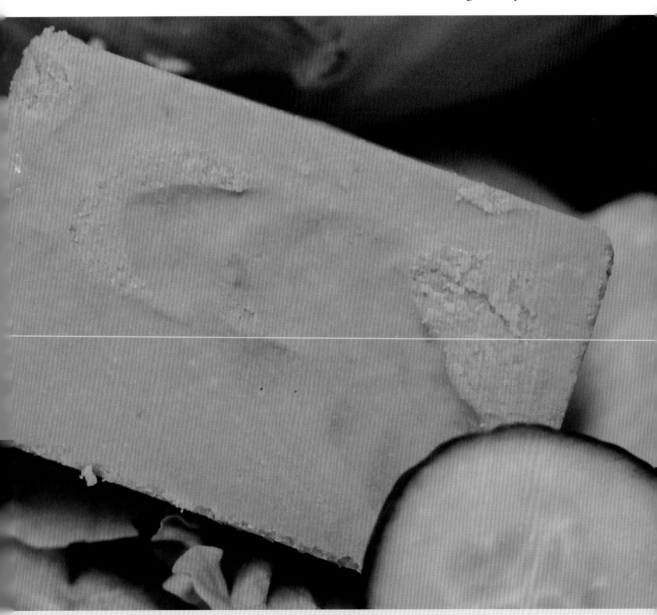

Pass the salad soap

Pumpkin pie soap

The perfect post-Halloween soap when you have pumpkin seeds and pumpkin flesh left over from your lanterns. If you can't find pumpkin seed oil, use olive oil instead. They both have the same SAP value so the recipe won't need adjusting if you simply swap one for the other. If you can't find a fresh pumpkin, use tinned pumpkin instead.

PUMPKIN PURÉE (BOIL UNTIL IT IS JUST TURNING SOFT)
30 g pumpkin flesh, cut into small cubes • 30 g water

LYE SOLUTION
138 g water • 64 g sodium hydroxide

SOAP OILS AND BUTTERS
250 g pumpkin seed oil • 150 g coconut oil • 50 g shea butter

SOAP SCENT
6 g pumpkin fragrance oil • 4 g blood orange essential oil
2 g ginger essential oil

ADDITIONS
Cleaned and baked pumpkin seeds (wash the seeds to remove pulp residue and lay out on a nonstick baking tray. Bake in a preheated oven at 200°C/400°F/Gas 6 for 10–15 minutes)

METHOD
Line your mould if necessary and place to one side.

Place the pumpkin cubes and 30 g water in a liquidiser; pulverise until you have a smooth purée.

Wearing safety equipment (page 10), make up your lye solution using 138 g water and 63 g sodium hydroxide. Set aside somewhere out of reach of children and pets.

Weigh the oils and butter and put them in a saucepan. Set the pan over a low heat until everything has melted.

Wearing safety goggles and gloves and paying careful attention to the safe handling of the lye (page 9), pour the lye into the mixture of butter and oils.

Stir briefly with a spoon to mix the oils, butter and lye together.

Add the pumpkin purée and blitz with a handheld stick blender until you have reached a light trace.

Add the fragrance oil and essential oils to the soap mixture and stir well.

Pour the soap mixture into your prepared mould. Sprinkle a handful of pumpkin seeds onto the surface of your soap.

Cover the mould with a lid, chopping board or a piece of cardboard to prevent the towels from falling into the soap. Now cover the covered mould with a layer of old towels and leave for 24 hours before removing from the mould.

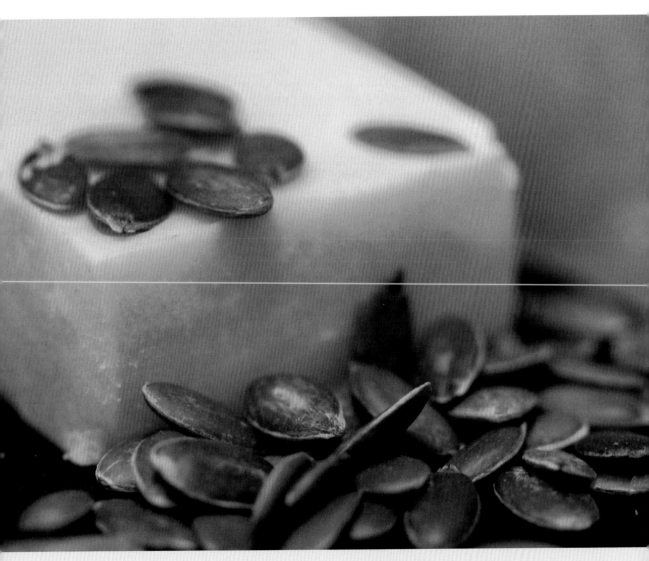

Pumpkin pie soap

Substituting the water in your lye

Once you've mastered the art of making soap you will start to become creative or even obsessed about what else you can include in your soaps. What better way of stretching the imagination than by substituting lye water for a different type of liquid instead?

There are many liquids that you can use as an alternative to water. The choice includes fruit juice, milk (cow's, goat's, buttermilk, coconut and breast milk), beer, wine, tea and coffee, but if you find something else you'd like to use it is probably perfectly possible to include it using one of the methods described here.

Because the liquids will be included with the sodium hydroxide as part of your lye solution, extra careful attention should be paid to the handling and creation of the lye, as the lye may be hotter and more active than usual.

Making milk soaps

You can include powdered milks in your soaps or you can add the milk in liquid form. Adding powdered milk is easier and since it is added at light trace, the lye is made up with sodium hydroxide and water as usual.

Using liquid milk in soaps is a great way of using up excess milk, though. If you wish to add milk in its liquid form then you will be adding it to the

Cow's milk soap

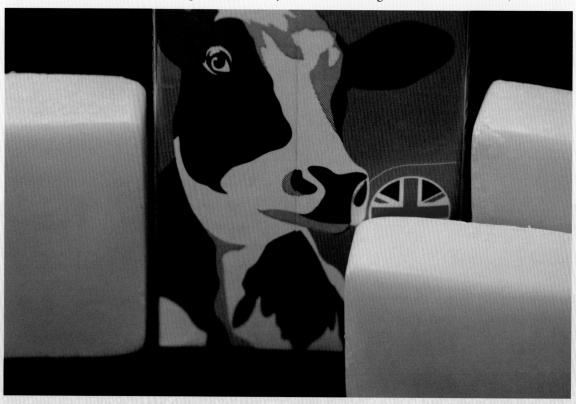

sodium hydroxide as part of your lye mixture. The lye may get hotter than usual and scald the milk. If you've ever smelt burnt milk then you will know that this isn't a particularly attractive aroma. The aroma won't translate through to the final bars of soap, but it will linger in your work area whilst you make the soap so open a window or two. Also, if the milk scalds, it turns the lye solution a shade of anything between bright orange to brown, which will have an impact on the final soap.

You can help to keep the lye cooler by placing water and ice cubes in the sink and standing your lye jug in the cold water. My preference for avoiding overheated lye is to freeze the milk before using it to make the lye. Please note that we don't advise superfatting your milk soaps (page 129) since the milk has a natural fat content itself. Adding excess oils on top of the milk may make your soaps greasy and will reduce the lathering capability. Milk soaps will have a shelf life of at least 18 months.

FREEZING YOUR MILK

To freeze your milk, you will need sets of ice-cube trays or small sealable freezer bags. With ice-cube trays, simply pour the milk into the compartments and place in the freezer until needed.

If you are using small sealable freezer bags you will find it easier to place a bag in a cup and fold the top of the bag over the edges of the cup to hold it in place. Pour the milk into the bag, squeeze as much air out of the bag as possible and seal it. Pop it into the freezer to freeze.

Frozen milk can remain fresh in the freezer for up to nine months.

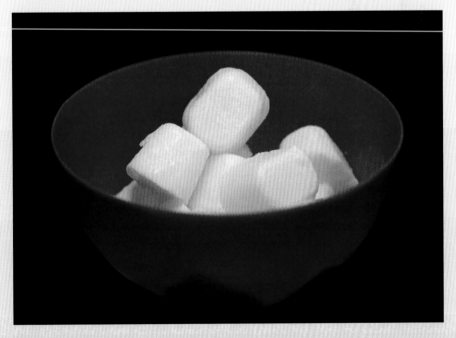

Frozen cubes of goats' milk from an ice-cube tray

TO GEL, OR NOT TO GEL?

During the 24-hour insulation period, soaps containing milk can get very hot, much hotter than the usual temperatures reached during the gel stage. This may not be a problem, but in some cases gelling can overheat your soap, causing the milk to burn and this in turn causes the soap to go brown, and possibly spoil. I found one block of soap had acted like boiling milk and had actually risen up and out of the soap mould. Rather than beautiful soap, I had a big mess to clear up!

To reduce the chances of this happening it may be better not to insulate your soap at all, but to simply leave it covered with a lid somewhere out of the way for 24 hours. There is a chance that the soap will attempt to gel, but will not be successful at gelling all the way through.

If a soap has started to gel, but not completed the gelling process to the very edges of the soap (gelling always starts in the centre of the soap, where it is at its warmest), you may find that the inner gelled part has a darker ring to the outside edges of the ungelled soap. The outside edges may also be a little crumbly and fall apart when you try to slice the soap. The soap is still perfectly okay to use, it just won't have the smooth sides you were hoping for.

REFRIGERATING YOUR SOAP

Another tip is to put your soap into the fridge for the first 24 hours. The cool temperatures will prevent the soap from gelling at all. It needn't only be milk soaps, any cold process soap can be kept in the fridge for the first 24 hours.

There are various advantages and disadvantages to placing your soap in the fridge, listed here below.

Advantages	Disadvantages
Milk soaps are less likely to burn	Soaps will take longer to firm up and the normal curing process is likely to be more like six weeks rather than four weeks
Milk soaps will retain their pale colour	Soaps may be a little softer than usual
Any fragrance or essential oil will hold its aroma better and for longer when the soap is brought back to room temperature	You may have difficulty getting your soap out of the mould initially as the soap will be a little moist. Leave it in the mould until it has hardened up and is therefore more easily removed

Softly, softly skin monkey soap

Milk is the perfect skin softener and it helps to make a very creamy bar. Here, we are making this recipe even more sumptuous by adding a little double cream.

Do make your lye solution up over the sink, so that any splashes or spillages from the over-active lye can be quickly and easily cleaned up. It goes without saying that wearing your protective gloves and mask are a must (page 10). If you are not using frozen milk, stand your lye jug in a sink of cold water and ice cubes and keep the milk in the fridge until you need to use it.

SOAP OILS AND BUTTERS
300 g olive oil • 100 g coconut oil • 50 g shea butter

LYE SOLUTION
168 g semi-skimmed or full-fat milk, chilled or frozen • 64 g sodium hydroxide

SOAP SCENT
12 g tonka bean fragrance oil

ADDITION
2 tablespoons double cream (pouring consistency)

METHOD
Line your mould if necessary and place to one side.

Weigh the oils and butter and put them into a saucepan. Set the pan over a low heat until everything has melted. Once melted, remove from the heat and leave somewhere to cool a little (actually, the cooler the better but you don't want the shea butter to start setting).

Weigh the sodium hydroxide and place safely to one side out of the reach of others.

Remove the milk from the fridge or freezer and place in a jug. Place the jug in the sink.

Slowly pour the sodium hydroxide into the milk. Stir to make sure the sodium hydroxide has dissolved. Do not be surprised if there is an ammonia-like aroma coming from the milk or if the lye changes colour.

Pour the lye into the cooled, melted oils and butter. Stir briefly with a spoon to mix the oils, butter and lye together.

Blitz with a handheld stick blender until you have reached a light trace. Add the tonka bean fragrance oil and double cream. Stir to ensure they are thoroughly mixed into the soap mixture.

Pour the soap mixture into your prepared mould. Cover the mould with a lid, chopping board or a piece of cardboard and place the soap in the fridge for at least 24 hours.

While the soap is hardening up, leave it in the mould and at room temperature. There is no need to insulate it at this time.

Once the soap is firm enough to remove from the mould (two to three weeks later), chop it into slices. You may find that as well as being softer, this soap is a little oilier than normal, so wipe away any oily residue and leave the soap a little longer than usual to harden up.

Leave the soap to cure at room temperature for at least six weeks before using it. Milk soaps are softer and require a longer curing time to harden up (most cold process soaps will harden nicely in four weeks). If you use them when they are still on the soft side, they will go mushy.

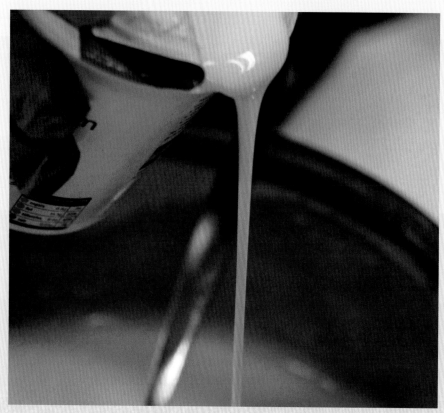

Pouring double cream into the soap at the light trace stage

Goats' milk with lemongrass

I strongly recommend that you use only frozen goats' milk to make up your lye to limit the heating and potential for scalding. Lemongrass blends beautifully with the goats' milk aroma.

SOAP OILS
50 g avocado oil • 250 g olive oil • 100 g coconut oil • 50 g palm oil

LYE SOLUTION
168 g frozen goats' milk • 65 g sodium hydroxide

SOAP SCENT
12 g lemongrass essential oil

COLOUR
Green CP colouring

METHOD
Line your mould if necessary and place to one side.

Weigh the oils and place them in a saucepan. Set the pan over a low heat until everything has melted. Once melted, remove from the heat and leave somewhere to cool a little.

Weigh the sodium hydroxide and place safely to one side out of the reach of others.

Remove your weighed goats' milk from the freezer and place in a jug. Place the jug in the sink.

Slowly pour the sodium hydroxide into the goats' milk. Stir to make sure the sodium hydroxide has dissolved. Do not be surprised if there is an ammonia-like aroma coming from the milk or if the lye changes colour.

Pour the lye into the cooled, melted oils. Stir briefly with a spoon to mix the oils and lye together.

Blitz with a handheld stick blender until you have reached a light trace. Add the lemongrass essential oil and stir until it has been thoroughly incorporated into the soap mixture.

Pour half of the soap mixture into the mould. Bang the mould onto your work surface firmly, once or twice, to remove any trapped air bubbles and to smooth out the surface of the soap.

Add the green CP colouring to the remaining soap and stir to blend it to a smooth mixture. Carefully pour this on top of the soap in the mould.

Cover the mould with a lid, chopping board or a piece of cardboard and place the soap in the fridge for at least 24 hours. Once the soap is firm enough to remove from the mould, chop into slices. This may take two or three weeks after making the soap. As with all milk-based soaps, leave the soap to cure at room temperature for at least six weeks before using it.

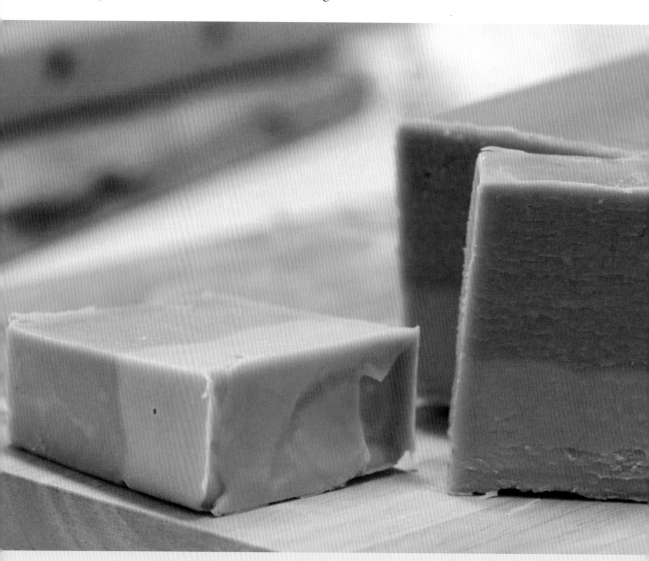

Goats' milk with lemongrass

Tropical coconut

In this soap I have selected coconut oil, coconut milk and coconut fragrance oil blended with lime. Enjoy a totally tropical, full-on coconut wash!

SOAP OILS AND BUTTERS
200 g coconut oil • 200 g olive oil • 50 g shea butter

LYE SOLUTION
168 g frozen coconut milk • 69 g sodium hydroxide

SOAP SCENT
6 g coconut fragrance oil • 6 g lime essential oil

METHOD
Line your mould if necessary and place to one side.

Weigh the oils and butter and place them into a saucepan. Set the pan over a low heat until everything has melted. Once melted, remove from the heat and leave somewhere to cool a little.

Weigh the sodium hydroxide and place safely to one side out of the reach of others.

Remove the weighed coconut milk from the freezer and place in a jug. Place the jug in the sink.

Slowly pour the sodium hydroxide into the coconut milk. Stir to make sure the sodium hydroxide has dissolved.

Pour the lye into the melted cooled oils and butter. Stir briefly with a spoon to mix the oils and lye together.

Blitz with a handheld stick blender until you have reached a light trace. Add the coconut fragrance oil with the lime essential oil and stir until thoroughly incorporated into the soap mixture.

Pour the soap mixture into the mould. Bang the mould onto your work surface to remove any trapped air bubbles and to smooth out the surface of the soap.

Cover the mould with a lid, chopping board or a piece of cardboard and place the soap in the fridge for at least 24 hours.

Once the soap is firm enough to remove from the mould, chop into slices. This may take up two or three weeks after making the soap. Leave the soap for at least six weeks to cure at room temperature before using it.

Tropical coconut soap

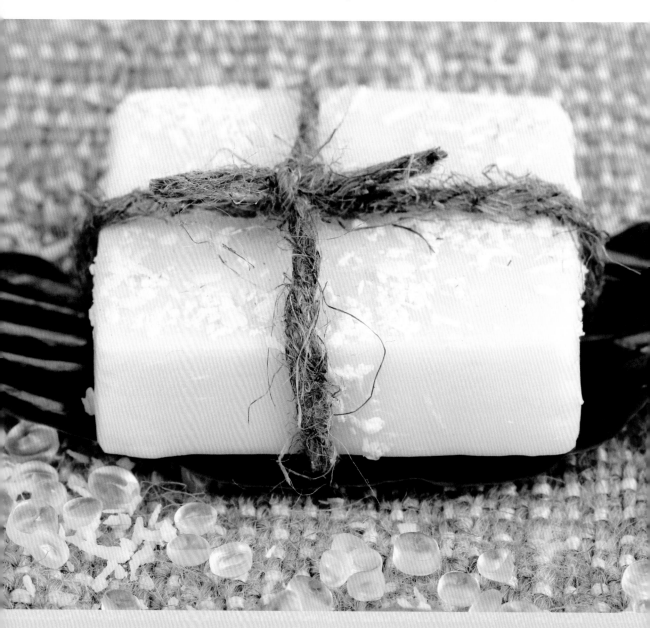

Rabi's sandalwood and buttermilk soap

This recipe was very kindly shared with us by Rabi, one of our lovely students in Nigeria. It uses sandalwood and buttermilk powders, which make the soap feel soft on your skin and they smell gorgeous! Forgive me, Rabi – I changed the smell a little, and have included sandalwood amyris essential oil, as it is more affordable.

Soap oils and butters
90 g sweet almond oil • 100 g fractionated coconut oil
300 g olive oil • 10 g shea butter

Lye solution
187 g water • 77 g sodium hydroxide

Additions
30 g buttermilk powder • 15 g sandalwood powder

Soap scent
10 g sandalwood amyris essential oil • 2 g ho wood essential oil

Method
Line your mould and place it to one side.

Make up your lye in the same way as the other recipes in this section and leave it somewhere safe to cool a little.

Weigh the oils and butter and place them in a saucepan. Set the pan over a low heat until everything has melted. Once melted, remove from the heat and add the lye solution.

Rabi's sandalwood and buttermilk soap

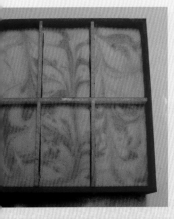

Bring your soap mixture to a light trace. Add the buttermilk powder and essential oils and stir well.

Take two tablespoons of the mixture out and place it in a small jug or bowl. Add the sandalwood powder to this and stir well.

Pour the uncoloured soap mixture into the mould and drizzle the sandalwood powder coloured mixture on top to create a swirled pattern.

Insulate and leave for 24 hours before slicing.

Making beer and wine soaps

Hops can have a soothing and anti-inflammatory effect on the skin, so what better way to apply them than in a bar of beer soap?

Before you embark on your soap making adventure please note that it is imperative that you use only flat, non-fizzy beer and wine. It is also important to remove the alcohol by cooking it off before you use it in your soap. Fizzy drinks and alcohol will cause the lye to react and make the soap seize and become too thick to manage effectively.

Any red, white, rosé or sparkling wine will do. Beers such as real ale, beer, lager and bière blonde can all be used provided they are no longer gassy. You can substitute all or part of the lye water with flat beer or wine.

Be prepared to work fast. Even though you will have cooked the alcohol out of the beers and wines, there is still a chance that it may accelerate and turn solid far more quickly than you were intending.

HOW TO PREPARE YOUR BEER FOR USE IN SOAP

In a large stainless steel saucepan, slowly bring the beer to a gentle boil and leave to boil for at least two minutes. Reduce the heat and simmer for a further five minutes before removing from the heat.

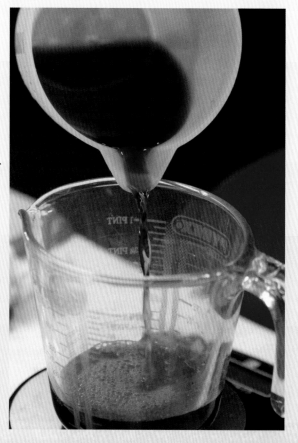

Using beer to make the lye

When the beer has cooled, pour into a smaller container and place it in the fridge until chilled.

Only now will the beer be suitable for use in soap. The alcohol will have been removed during the cooking process and the entire cooking and cooling process encourages the beer to go flat.

The flat beer will remain good to use in soap for at least two weeks if you keep it in a lidded container in the fridge. Beer soaps will have a shelf life of at least two years.

ESSENTIAL AND FRAGRANCE OILS TO USE IN BEER SOAPS

Your soap will have a natural stale beer aroma, which may not be what you were expecting and I should think probably not what you were hoping for either! Select essential or fragrance oils that blend well with the smell of beer to give a more pleasing aroma.

Whilst it is purely down to personal preference, there are a few certain oils that we have found work particularly well.

ESSENTIAL OILS IN BEER SOAPS

Whilst citrus oils don't hold their aroma too well in traditional soaps, the blend of beer, barley, wheat, hops and citrus works well and it is definitely worth trying. Lime (think along the lines of Mexican cerveza beer that is served with a wedge of lime pushed into the neck of the bottle), orange, mandarin and lemon are my particular favourites.

Essential oils with a spicy edge blend nicely with the smell of beer, barley and hops. Aniseed (which reminds me of a liquorice-type root beer), ginger (as in ginger beer), cloves and a little cinnamon all work well. Even though I'm not a huge fan of chamomile, it has a grassy, hay-like thread that blends well with the soapy hop smell.

Woody essential oils are always a safe bet, especially as it is highly likely that your beer soaps will appeal to men and men are easily drawn to the woody aromas. Try patchouli

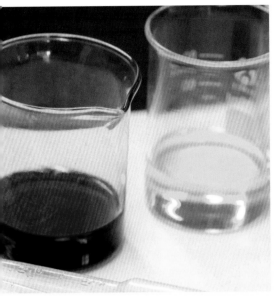

Choose essential oils that will work with the natural aroma of the beer

and vetiver or amyris essential oils.

There are an abundance of fragrance oils that will enhance the aroma of your beer soaps, such as honey, oakmoss, vanilla, chocolate and even some of the fruity fragrances like strawberry, raspberry, blackcurrant and cherry. Failing that, you can actually get fragrance oils that smell of beer, barley or hops. The Guinness soap overleaf could be made even more authentic with the inclusion of Guinness fragrance oil.

BEER SOAP RECIPES

The beer soaps could easily be created using the hot process or slow cooker (crock-pot) methods, but to keep things simple, we're using the cold process method. Feel free to choose whichever method you prefer.

Before starting to make these soaps, prepare the beer by boiling, simmering and cooling it. This will have to be done at least a day ahead of making your soap. The natural colour of your soaps will be brown, which coincidentally is pretty much the same colour as most beers so no need to add colour unless you want a coloured effect. That said, since Guinness is black we coloured that soap black with a creamy coloured head.

HANDLING BEER LYE

Please make sure that you adhere to all the safety guidelines and wear your safety glasses and gloves (page 10) when working with beer. Lye made with beer rather than water can behave like a beast! Place your lye jug in an empty sink so that if there is any unwanted activity or lye volcano, you are well placed to flush any spillage down the sink.

MAKING STRONG WATER LYE WITH A BEER TOP UP

If you are concerned about mixing sodium hydroxide with the beer then make a strong, water version of the lye first. To do this, make up your lye using sodium hydroxide and 100 g water and stir until the sodium hydroxide has dissolved. Now top up the lye with 68 g cold, flat beer to make 168 g liquid in total.

SOAP RECIPES USING BEER

Apart from the ideas given here, any of the soap recipes in this book can be converted to beer soaps simply by substituting all or some of the lye water with cool, flat beer. Have fun experimenting to perfect your own versions.

Please see the more detailed description of making cold process soap in the soap making methods section (pages 37–8) as I have only included an abridged version here.

My Guinness, my goodness!

Lovely dark, rich, iconic Guinness makes a beautiful soap. Guinness beer is so dark that it appears almost black in its glass, but sports a glorious cream coloured head. Here, our Guinness soap tries to emulate the black and cream colour scheme.

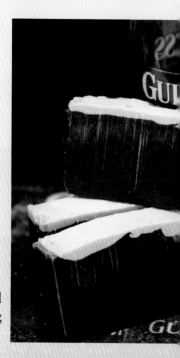

LYE SOLUTION
168 g flat, cold Guinness (or use a combination of Guinness and water, provided it weighs 168 g in total) • 62 g sodium hydroxide

SOAP OILS AND BUTTERS
50 g castor oil • 235 g olive oil • 100 g coconut oil • 50 g cocoa butter

SOAP SCENT
6 g aniseed essential oil • 3 g chamomile essential oil
3 g coffee fragrance oil

COLOURS
5 g titanium dioxide (mixed with 10 g olive oil for a slurry)
5 g black oxide (mixed with 10 g olive oil to create a slurry)

METHOD
Prepare your equipment and mould.

Weigh the cold, flat Guinness and sodium hydroxide. Place your weighed Guinness in a jug and stand the jug in the sink. If you prefer to use the strong water lye with a beer top up, see the instructions at the top of this page.

Carefully tip the sodium hydroxide into the cold, flat Guinness, then stir until the sodium hydroxide has dissolved. Do not worry if the colour and the aroma of the lye are unpleasant at this stage. Set your lye jug aside somewhere safe.

Weigh the soap oils and butter and put into a stainless steel saucepan. Set over a low heat until melted together. Remove the saucepan from the heat.

Pour a small amount of the lye into the melted oils to make sure there is no adverse fizzing reaction. If there is a reaction, wait until the oils and lye have cooled slightly before continuing. If no reaction, pour the rest of the Guinness lye into the melted oils.

Using a handheld stick blender, mix the oils and lye together until they form a light trace.

Add the essential and fragrance oils and stir to make sure that these have been thoroughly incorporated into your soap.

Pour one third of the scented soap mixture into a jug and – working fairly quickly – add the white titanium slurry and mix well.

Again, working quickly, add the black oxide slurry to the soap in the saucepan and mix well.

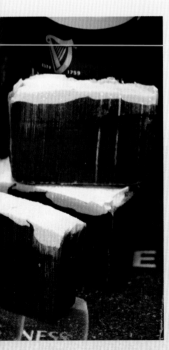

Pour the darker portion of the soap into the prepared mould. Bang the mould onto a work surface to knock out any air bubbles and to smooth the surface of the soap. Carefully pour the paler portion of the soap mixture on top of the darker portion being careful not to dislodge the smooth surface of the dark soap. You may find it easier to first pour the soap onto a spatula held just about the darker portion.

Please note: if your mould is upside down and therefore the first portion of soap poured in becomes the top of your soap, you will have to pour the other way round. If this is the case, pour the lighter coloured soap in first and then pour the darker soap on top.

Cover the mould and insulate for the next 24 hours (see step 10 on page 38) before removing the soap from the mould and leaving to cure at room temperature.

My Guinness, my goodness! soap

Real ale nut butter bar

Hazelnut oil and hazelnut fragrance oil give this soap a nutty aroma that teams well with the beer. I have chosen to use cold, flat London Pride by Fuller's Brewery, but you could easily replace it with another real ale – perhaps one local to where you live?

LYE SOLUTION
168 g flat, cold London Pride (or use a combination of London Pride/water provided it weighs 168 g in total) • 58 g sodium hydroxide

SOAP OILS AND BUTTERS
200 g hazelnut oil • 150 g olive oil • 100 g shea butter

SOAP SCENT
12 g hazelnut fragrance oil

COLOUR
2 g black oxide (combine with 5 g water to make a slurry)

METHOD
Prepare your equipment and mould.

Weigh the London Pride beer and sodium hydroxide. Place your weighed beer in a jug and stand the jug in the sink. If you prefer to use the strong water lye with a beer top up, please see the instructions at the beginning of the beer recipes (page 98) and then continue weighing the oils.

Carefully tip the sodium hydroxide into the beer and stir until it has dissolved. Do not worry if the colour and the aroma of the beer lye are unpleasant at this stage. Set your lye jug aside somewhere safe.

Weigh the oils and butter and put them into a stainless steel saucepan. Place over a low heat until the solid oils and butter have melted. Remove the saucepan from the heat.

Pour a small amount of the lye into the melted oils to make sure there is no adverse fizzing reaction. If there is a reaction, wait until the oils and lye have cooled slightly before continuing. If no reaction, pour the rest of the real ale lye into the melted oils.

Using a handheld stick blender, mix the oils and lye together until they form a light trace.

Add the hazelnut fragrance oil and stir to make sure that it is thoroughly incorporated into your soap.

Remove approximately 6 tablespoons of the soap and put into a small container. Add the black oxide slurry and mix well.

Pour the uncoloured soap into the prepared mould. Bang the mould onto a work surface to knock out any air bubbles and to smooth the surface of the soap. Drizzle the black oxide slurry onto the soap and carefully create a pattern by swirling or dragging using the tip of a teaspoon handle.

Cover the mould and insulate for the next 24 hours (see step 10 on page 38) before removing the soap from the mould and leaving to cure at room temperature.

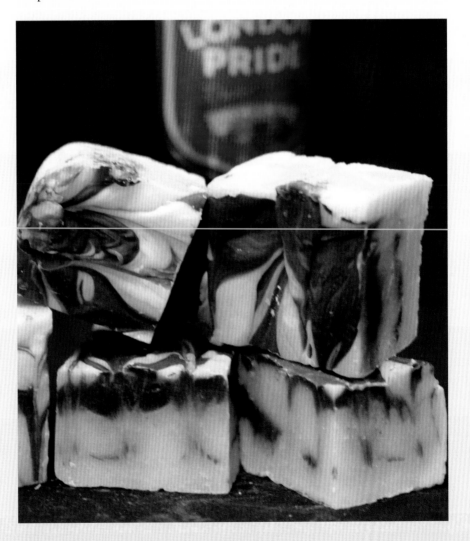

Real ale nut butter bar

IPA bars for Jake Bugg

First, I fell in love with the song, then I fell in love with singer-songwriter Jake Bugg. If you have no idea what I'm talking about, google the Greene King IPA advert! It conjures up a feel-good, friendly, typically English pub and has the lovely, gravelly-voiced Jake Bugg singing a gentle country song throughout. Whilst I don't tend to drink IPA, I did rush out and buy Jake Bugg's CD, which I can highly recommend. Even though I doubt he will ever read this book, let alone make his own soap, this recipe is dedicated to him as a thank you.

LYE SOLUTION
168 g cold, flat IPA (or use a combination of IPA and water provided it weighs 168 g in total) • 63 g sodium hydroxide

SOAP OILS AND BUTTERS
150 g olive oil • 100 g coconut oil • 50 g palm oil
100 g rice bran oil • 50 g shea butter

SOAP SCENT
6 g patchouli essential oil • 3 g vetiver essential oil
3 g mandarin essential oil mixed together with 15 g argan oil (something special for you, Jake!)

METHOD
Prepare your equipment and mould.

Weigh your cold, flat IPA and sodium hydroxide. Place your weighed beer in a jug and stand the jug in the sink. If you prefer to use the strong water lye with a beer top up, please see the instructions at the beginning of the beer recipes (page 98) and then continue from weighing the oils.

Carefully tip the sodium hydroxide into the beer and stir until the sodium hydroxide has dissolved (do not worry if the colour and the aroma of the beer lye are unpleasant at this stage). Set your lye jug aside somewhere safe.

Weigh the oils and butter and put into a stainless steel saucepan. Place over a low heat until they have melted together. Remove the saucepan from the heat.

Pour a small amount of lye into the melted oils and butter to make sure there is no adverse fizzing reaction. If there is a reaction, wait until the oils and lye have cooled slightly before continuing. If not, pour the rest of the IPA lye into the mixture of melted oils and butter.

Using a handheld stick blender, mix the oils and lye together until they form a light trace.

Add the essential oils blended in argan oil and stir to make sure that they have been thoroughly incorporated into your soap.

Pour the soap into the prepared mould. Bang the mould onto a work surface to knock out any air bubbles and to smooth the surface of the soap.

Cover the mould and insulate for the next 24 hours (page 38) before removing the soap from the mould and leaving to cure at room temperature.

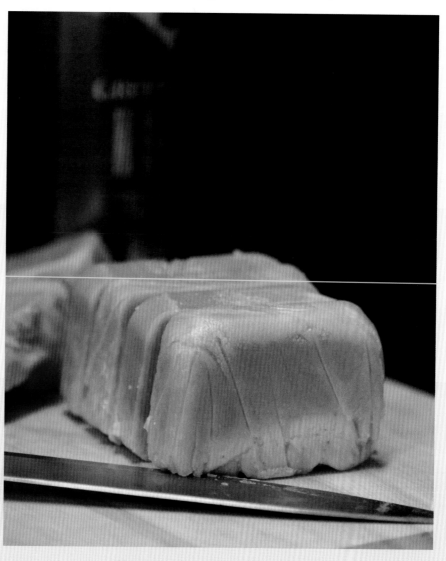

IPA bars inspired by and dedicated to Jake Bugg

Muchas gracias cerveza soap

A lighter soap made with lager rather than beer and, in true Mexican style, I've added a twist of lime.

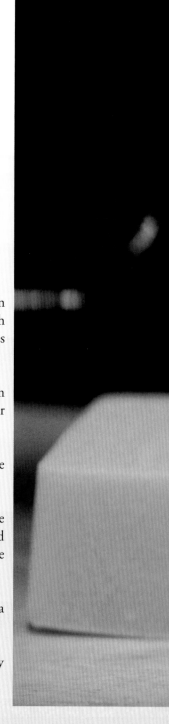

LYE SOLUTION
168 g cold, flat lager
(or use a combination of lager and water provided it weighs 168 g in total)
62 g sodium hydroxide

SOAP OILS AND BUTTERS
100 g sweet almond oil • 100 g apricot kernel oil
100 g avocado oil • 100 g coconut oil • 50 g shea butter

SOAP SCENT
12 g lime essential oil

METHOD
Prepare your equipment and mould.

Weigh your cold, flat lager and sodium hydroxide. Place your weighed lager in a jug and stand the jug in the sink. If you prefer to use the strong water lye with a lager top up, please see the instructions at the beginning of the beer recipes (page 98) and then continue from weighing the oils and butter.

Carefully tip the sodium hydroxide into the lager and stir until the sodium hydroxide has dissolved (do not worry if the colour and the aroma of the lager lye are unpleasant at this stage). Set your lye jug aside somewhere safe.

Weigh the oils and butter and put them into a stainless steel saucepan. Place over a low heat until melted together. Remove the saucepan from the heat.

Pour a small amount of lye into the melted oils to make sure there is no adverse fizzing reaction. If there is a reaction, wait until the oils and lye have cooled slightly before continuing. If no reaction, pour the rest of the lager lye into the melted oils.

Using a handheld stick blender, mix the oils and lye together until they form a light trace.

Add the lime essential oil and stir to make sure that this has been thoroughly incorporated into your soap.

Muchas gracias
cerveza soap

Cover the mould and insulate for the next 24 hours (see page 38) before removing the soap from the mould and leaving to cure at room temperature.

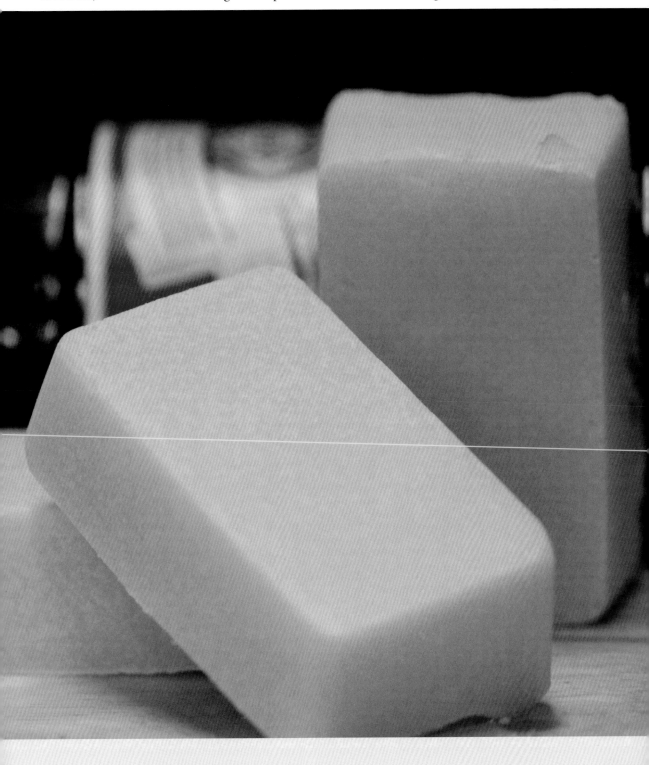

HOW TO PREPARE YOUR WINE FOR USE IN SOAP

Red and white wine are not naturally fizzy, so whilst it is important to remove the alcohol, there is no fizz to remove. However, if you plan to use champagne or sparkling wines in your soap then sadly the fizz must go.

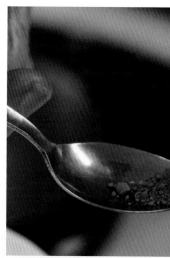

For all types of wine, slowly bring to a gentle boil and leave to boil for at least two minutes. Reduce the heat and simmer for a further five minutes to remove all traces of alcohol before removing it from the heat.

When the wine has cooled, pour it into a smaller container and place in the fridge until it is chilled. Only now will the wine be suitable for use in soap. The alcohol will have been removed during the cooking process and the entire cooking and cooling process encourages any fizz to go flat.

If you do not first cook the alcohol out of the red and white wine, when you include these in your soap, the alcohol content will cause the soap to seize and go very thick extremely quickly. This may be too thick even to blend in your fragrance and essential oils.

The flat wines will remain good to use in soap for at least two weeks if you keep them in a lidded container in the fridge. Wine soaps have a shelf life of at least two years.

ESSENTIAL AND FRAGRANCE OILS TO USE IN WINE SOAPS

In this case your soap will have a natural wine-in-lye aroma that isn't at all agreeable. You will definitely want to add fragrance or essential oils to mask the natural aroma. Choosing the aromas to use is made easy for you. When reading any description of wine you will find that many of the words used to describe it will match essential or fragrance oils that you hopefully already have in your collection. For example, the words used to describe many light, dry white wines include apple, apricot, citrus, peach, spice and floral, whilst some chardonnays are described using words such as butter, popcorn, vanilla and honey. I see on the label of my sauvignon blanc that I should be able to detect the flavours of citrus notes (lemon, lime and grapefruit), summer fruit (peach, nectarine, apricot, papaya), fresh cut grass, sweet peas, smoke and gooseberry. Red wines are typically heavy and you'll need a selection of more robust fragrance and essential oils, such as cherries, berries, vanilla, chocolate, raisins, oak, liquorice, plum and tobacco.

There you see – all you need is Google and a friendly wine merchant and you'll easily be able to find out what kind of fragrance and essential oil you can use to enhance your wine soaps. But if in doubt, use grape fragrance oil.

COLOURING WINE SOAPS

The beer soaps turn a shade of brown, which is more than suitable as beers themselves are mostly brown. Red, white and champagne soaps will also turn a

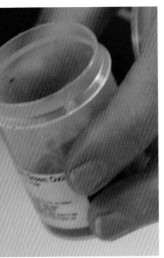

Using green oxide to colour a white wine soap mixture

shade of brown which is less becoming. To counteract the natural brown you will need colours that can bring the soap back to something more in keeping with the natural wine colour.

For red wine, a bordeaux or autumn red coloured mica works well. Red oxide is a little too 'brick-dust' in colour and therefore unsuitable as a shade of wine.

For white wine soaps I suggest that you use a green oxide or mica such as mermaid or sea green or the liquid CP colour. Whilst white wine is usually pale golden, the grapes are green as are the bottles so the overall effect, even with the tinge of brown, will veer towards green.

It is not so simple for champagne soaps as trying to get a pale golden colour when the soap naturally turns a shade of brown is very difficult. I suggest that you stick with the drinking theme and perhaps include your champagne as part of a 'Bucks Fizz' soap and colour and fragrance it orange, or a 'Kir Royal', making the soap darker red and including blackcurrant as the fragrance. There's a whole range of champagne cocktails and I suggest you use them as inspiration for your champagne soaps.

HANDLING WINE LYE

Please make sure that you adhere to all the safety guidelines and wear your safety glasses and gloves (page 10). Like beer soaps, lye made with wine rather than water can be quite volatile. Place your lye jug in an empty sink so that if there is a lye volcano, you are well placed to flush the spillage down the sink.

MAKING STRONG WATER LYE WITH A WINE TOP-UP

If you are concerned about mixing sodium hydroxide with wine then please make a strong, water version of the lye first. To do this, make up your lye using sodium hydroxide and 100 g water; stir until the sodium hydroxide has dissolved. Now top up the lye with 68 g cooked, cooled wine to make 168 g liquid in total.

Apart from the ideas given here, any of the soap recipes in this book can be converted to wine soaps simply by substituting all or some of the lye water with cooked, cooled wine. Please see the more detailed description of making cold process soap found in the soap making methods section (pages 37–8) as I have only included an abridged version here.

SOAP RECIPES USING WINE

Although these recipes make the wine soaps using the cold process method, you could choose to use the hot process or slow cooker (crock-pot) method instead.

Before starting to make any of the wine soaps, prepare your wine by boiling, simmering and cooling it. This will need to be done at least one day ahead of your soap making session.

Merlot mango mania

It's not often that we have any merlot left over to make soap so for me, the most difficult part of this recipe is finding a bottle that I'm happy to part with. Don't use an expensive wine since cheap and cheerful varieties will produce just as good soap. Save the pricier bottles for drinking rather than soaping!

LYE SOLUTION
168 g cooked, cooled merlot red wine
(or use a combination of wine and water provided it weighs 168 g in total)
63 g sodium hydroxide

SOAP OILS AND BUTTERS
100 g coconut oil • 250 g olive oil • 100 g mango butter

SOAP SCENT
9 g mango fragrance oil • 3 g plum fragrance oil

COLOUR
1–2 teaspoons bordeaux red mica (mix with 10 g water to create a slurry)

METHOD
Prepare your equipment and mould.

Measure the cooked, cooled wine and sodium hydroxide. Place your wine in a jug and stand it in the sink. If you prefer to use the strong water lye with a merlot top up, please see the instructions at the beginning of the wine recipes (page 107) and then continue from weighing the oils and butter.

Carefully tip the sodium hydroxide into the merlot and stir until the sodium hydroxide has dissolved (do not worry if the colour and the aroma of the wine lye are unpleasant at this stage). Set your lye jug aside somewhere safe.

Weigh the oils and butter and put them in a stainless steel saucepan. Place over a low heat until melted together. Remove the saucepan from the heat.

Pour a small amount of lye into the melted oils to make sure there is no adverse fizzing reaction. If there is a reaction, wait until the oils and lye have cooled slightly before continuing. If there is no reaction, pour the rest of the wine lye into the melted oils.

Using a handheld stick blender, mix the oils and lye together until they form a light trace.

Add the mango and plum fragrance oils and stir to make sure that this has been thoroughly incorporated into your soap.

Add the bordeaux red oxide slurry to your soap and mix well.

Pour the soap into the prepared mould. Bang the mould onto the work surface to knock out any air bubbles and to smooth the surface of the soap.

Cover the mould and insulate for the next 24 hours (see page 38) before removing the soap from the mould and leaving to cure at room temperature.

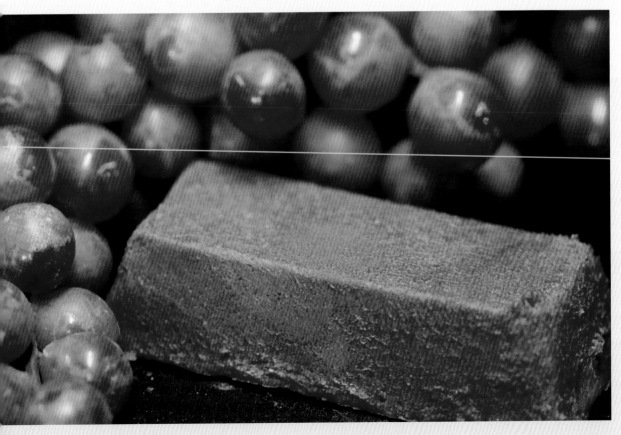

Merlot mango mania soap

Blackberry and elderflower wine soap

Hedgerow soaps are always popular and although this one has no actual botanicals in it, it remains a firm favourite.

LYE SOLUTION
168 g cooked, cooled red wine
(or use a combination of wine and water provided it weighs 168 g in total)
58 g sodium hydroxide

SOAP OILS AND BUTTERS
200 g olive oil • 100 g palm oil • 100 g rice bran oil • 50 g cocoa butter

SOAP SCENT
6 g blackberry fragrance oil • 3 g plum fragrance oil
3 g elderflower fragrance oil

COLOURS
1–2 teaspoons autumn red mica (mix with 10 g water to create a slurry)
$^1/_2$ teaspoon purple mica (mix with 5 g water for a slurry)

METHOD
Prepare your equipment and mould.

Weigh the cooked, cooled red wine and sodium hydroxide. Place your weighed red wine in a jug and stand the jug in the sink. If you prefer to use the strong water lye with a red wine top up, please see the instructions at the beginning of the wine recipes (page 98) and then continue from weighing the oils and butter.

Carefully tip the sodium hydroxide into the red wine and stir until the sodium hydroxide has dissolved (do not worry if the colour and the aroma of the wine lye are unpleasant at this stage). Set your lye jug aside somewhere safe.

Weigh the oils and butter and put into a stainless steel saucepan. Place over a low heat until melted together. Remove the saucepan from the heat.

Pour a small amount of lye into the melted oils to make sure there is no adverse fizzing reaction. If there is a reaction, wait until the oils and lye have cooled slightly before continuing. If no reaction, pour the rest of the wine lye into the melted oils.

Using a handheld stick blender, mix the oils and lye together until they form a light trace.

Add the blackberry, plum and elderflower fragrance oils; stir to make sure that they are thoroughly incorporated into your soap.

Pour one third of the soap mixture into the mould.

Add the autumn red slurry to the remaining soap mixture and stir well. Pour half of the mixture onto the uncoloured mixture in the soap mould.

Add the purple mica slurry to the final third left in the saucepan and stir well. Carefully pour this layer onto the other two layers in the mould.

Cover the mould and insulate for the next 24 hours (see page 38) before removing from the mould and leaving to cure at room temperature.

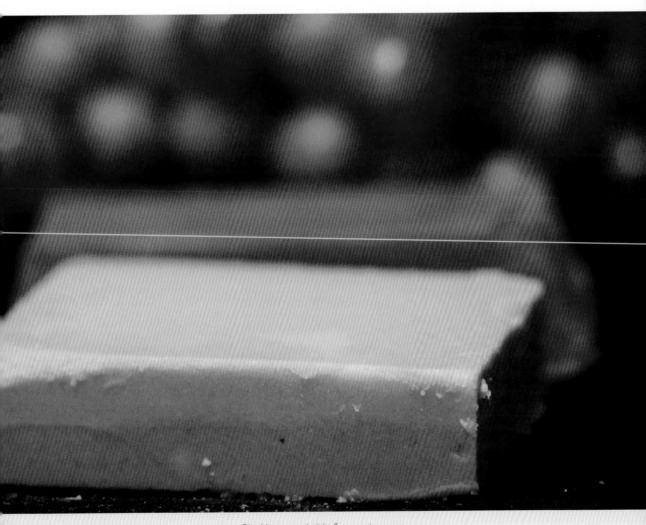

Blackberry and elderflower wine soap

Prosecco and gooseberry crush

If you choose an aroma that is predominately green, no one will ever question your prosecco soap being green rather than golden. The gooseberry fragrance oil is tart and crisp and the perfect aroma for this soap. If you can't find gooseberry fragrance oil, a good substitute is green apple fragrance oil mixed with a little lemon essential oil.

Lye solution
168 g cooked, cooled prosecco
(or use a combination of prosecco and water provided it weighs 168 g in total)
65 g sodium hydroxide

Soap oils
150 g olive oil • 150 g coconut oil • 150 g sweet almond oil

Soap scent
12 g gooseberry fragrance oil

Colour
1 teaspoon mermaid green mica (mix with 5 g water to create a slurry)

Method
Prepare your equipment and mould.

Weigh your cooked, cooled prosecco and sodium hydroxide. Place the weighed wine in a jug and stand the jug in the sink. If you prefer to use the strong water lye with a white wine top up, please see the instructions at the beginning of the wine recipes (page 98) and then continue from weighing the oils.

Carefully tip the sodium hydroxide into the wine and stir until the sodium hydroxide has dissolved (do not worry if the colour and the aroma of the wine lye are unpleasant at this stage). Set your lye jug aside somewhere safe.

Weigh the oils and put into a stainless steel saucepan. Place over a low heat until melted together. Remove the saucepan from the heat.

Pour a small amount of lye into the melted oils to make sure there is no adverse fizzing reaction. If there is a reaction, wait until the oils and lye have cooled slightly before continuing. If no reaction, pour the rest of the wine lye into the melted oils.

Using a handheld stick blender, mix the oils and lye together until they form a light trace.

Add the gooseberry fragrance oil and stir to make sure that it has been thoroughly incorporated into your soap.

Remove about one third of the soap mixture and colour it with the green mica slurry.

Pour half the uncoloured soap into the mould. Bang the mould onto the work surface to remove any trapped air bubbles.

Pour the green soap over the uncoloured soap and then pour the remaining uncoloured soap on top of the green layer.

Cover the mould and insulate for the next 24 hours (see page 38) before removing from the mould and leaving to cure at room temperature.

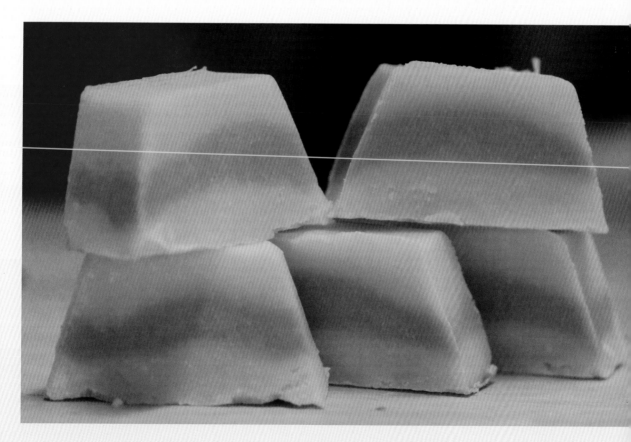

Prosecco and gooseberry crush soap

Post-party blues

The first champagne soap I ever made was after a post-party clear up when not-quite-empty bottles of champagne had been left out overnight. The fizz had naturally disappeared and whilst the flat champagne wasn't worth drinking, I simply could not bring myself to throw it away. So, of course, I used it in soap!

Whilst champagne isn't blue, I have put a little blue into the soap just to emphasise the morning-after-the-night-before 'blue' post-party mood.

LYE SOLUTION
165 g cooked, cooled, flat champagne (or use a combination of flat champagne and water provided it weighs 165 g in total)
54 g sodium hydroxide

SOAP OILS AND BUTTERS
100 g castor oil • 50 g jojoba oil • 200 g olive oil
50 g rice bran oil • 50 g rosehip oil

SOAP SCENT
12 g rose geranium essential oil

COLOUR
2 teaspoons blue ultramarine (mix with 25 g water to create a slurry)

METHOD
Prepare your equipment and mould.

Weigh your cooked, cooled, flat champagne and sodium hydroxide. Place the champagne in a jug and stand the jug in the sink. If you prefer to use the strong water lye with a flat champagne top up, please see the instructions at the beginning of the wine recipes (page 98) and then continue from weighing the oils.

Carefully tip the sodium hydroxide into the champagne wine and stir until the sodium hydroxide has dissolved (do not worry if the colour and the aroma of the champagne lye are unpleasant at this stage). Set your lye jug aside somewhere safe.

Weigh the oils and put into a stainless steel saucepan or large plastic container. Since these are all liquid oils there is no need to heat them.

Pour the champagne lye into the oils and stir.

Using a handheld stick blender, mix the oils and lye together until they form a light trace.

Add the rose geranium essential oil and stir to make sure that it has been thoroughly incorporated into your soap.

Pour a third of the soap mixture into a jug. Add one teaspoon of the blue ultramarine slurry and mix well. Pour the blue soap mixture into a mould. Bang the mould onto the work surface to remove any trapped air bubbles and to smooth the top of the soap.

Pour another third of the soap mixture into a jug. Add two teaspoons of the blue ultramarine slurry and mix well. Pour this slightly darker blue soap mixture into the mould on top of the lighter blue layer. Gently tap the mould onto the work surface to remove any trapped air bubbles and to smooth the top of the soap.

Add the last three teaspoons of the blue ultramarine slurry into the last third of the uncoloured soap mixture and stir well. Gently pour the darkest blue soap mixture into the mould on top of the other two blue layers. Tap the mould on the work surface to remove any trapped air bubbles and to smooth the top of the soap.

Cover the mould and insulate for the next 24 hours (see page 38) before removing the soap from the mould and leaving to cure at room temperature.

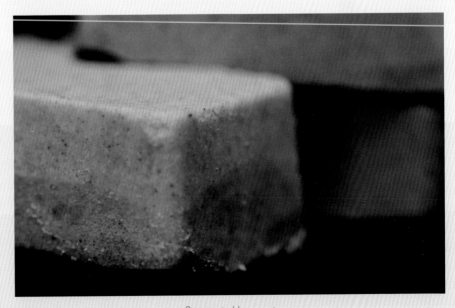

Post-party blues soap

Summer lemonade cup soap

Last, but by no means least, as I'm sure you will be creating similar soap recipes, we finish our alcohol section with a typically English summer drink. Pimm's is an alcoholic summer cordial that requires diluting with lemonade or tonic water. Usually the drink is served with pieces of cucumber, strawberry and apple and a sprig of mint. I rose to the challenge set by my lovely friend Ruth and came up with a soap version of this refreshing drink. If you can't get hold of Pimm's, you could replace it with gin. This recipe combines melt-and-pour soap with cold process soap, since I have embedded little strawberry-shaped and scented red melt-and-pour soaps into the cold process soap. It works best if you use individual moulds rather than the loaf type.

Before making this recipe you must make sure that all the alcohol has been cooked out of the Pimm's (or gin) just as for wine (page 106) and that the fizz has been removed from the lemonade. It is possible just to leave the lemonade to go flat, but as you need to cook the Pimm's anyway, you might as well cook the lemonade at the same time. This will definitely remove any fizz.

FOR THE STRAWBERRY MELT-AND-POUR SOAPS
100 g clear melt-and-pour soap base
A few drops of red liquid colouring • 2 g strawberry fragrance oil

LYE SOLUTION
30 g Pimm's • 138 g lemonade • 62 g sodium hydroxide

SOAP OILS AND BUTTERS
80 g coconut oil • 70 g palm oil • 250 g olive oil • 50 g shea butter

SOAP SCENT
10 g cucumber fragrance oil • 2 g spearmint (garden mint) essential oil

METHOD
Melt the clear melt-and-pour soap base (page 170) and add the red colouring and strawberry fragrance oil. Stir well and pour into small, strawberry shaped moulds – an ice-cube tray with little strawberry shaped cavities is perfect. Leave to set before removing from the mould. Place the little strawberry shaped soaps in the freezer.

Prepare your equipment and mould for the body of the soap.

Weigh your cooked, cooled Pimm's and lemonade mixture and sodium hydroxide. Place the Pimm's and lemonade in a jug and stand it in the sink.

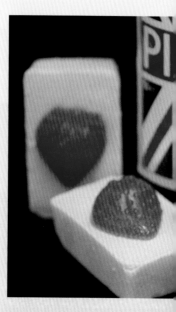

Carefully tip the sodium hydroxide into the Pimm's and lemonade and stir until the sodium hydroxide has dissolved (do not worry if the colour and the aroma of the Pimm's lye are unpleasant at this stage). Set your lye jug aside somewhere safe.

Weigh the oils and butter and put them into a stainless steel saucepan. Place over a low heat until melted together. Remove the saucepan from the heat and leave to cool for five minutes.

Pour a small amount of lye into the melted oils to make sure there is no adverse fizzing reaction. If there is a reaction, wait until the oils and lye have cooled slightly before continuing. If no reaction, pour the rest of the Pimm's and lemonade lye into the melted oils and butter.

Using a handheld stick blender, mix the oils and lye together until they form a light trace.

Add the cucumber and mint oil blend and stir to make sure that this has been thoroughly incorporated into your soap.

Pour the soap into the individual soap moulds.

Remove the strawberry soaps from the freezer and carefully insert them into the Pimm's soap so that they are lying on top of each bar. You will have far more success in doing this if the Pimm's soap has started to set a little.

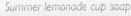

Summer lemonade cup soap

Pop the moulds into the fridge for 24 hours. Once the soaps are out of the fridge and removed from the moulds, they will need to be left for the usual four weeks to cure at room temperature.

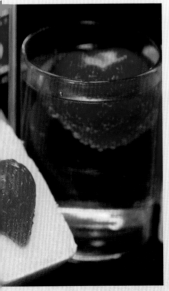

Making honey soaps

Honey is such a popular ingredient in soap. Depending on the soap making stage at which you include the honey, you may not require any additional aroma, since it can impart a glorious caramel honey fragrance of its own.

Honey can be added in the lye or at trace and will behave a little differently according to when it is added. Adding honey to the lye will cause it to burn and turn the lye solution brown. Burnt honey takes on the aroma of caramel, which gives your soap a beautiful and natural scent, but it will also discolour the soap.

If you want to keep the soap as pale as possible then I suggest that you add the honey at trace. Because the honey is not then cooked by the lye, its aroma is kept to a minimum, allowing you to use other fragrance or essential oils to scent your soap.

Each of the recipes described here will work equally well whether you add your honey to the lye or to the traced soap mixture so do feel free to switch methods to whichever you prefer.

You can choose to leave the soap somewhere at room temperature for the first 24 hours. Cover with only one layer of towels since the soap will become naturally hotter than usual due to the honey content. You may choose to put the soap in the fridge instead of leaving it under a towel.

Honey also works well in a hot process soap (see pages 47–9).

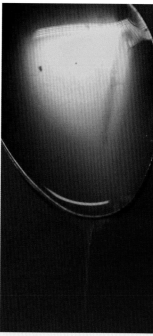

Honey can add colour, aroma and skin softness to your soap

SOAP RECIPES USING HONEY

Honey can easily be included in your soaps and will add extra moisturising and skin-softening properties. It will impart a subtle honeyed-caramel aroma which can be topped up by the addition of honey fragrance oil or other sweet fragrances.

Adding honey to your lye produces a dark caramel fragrance

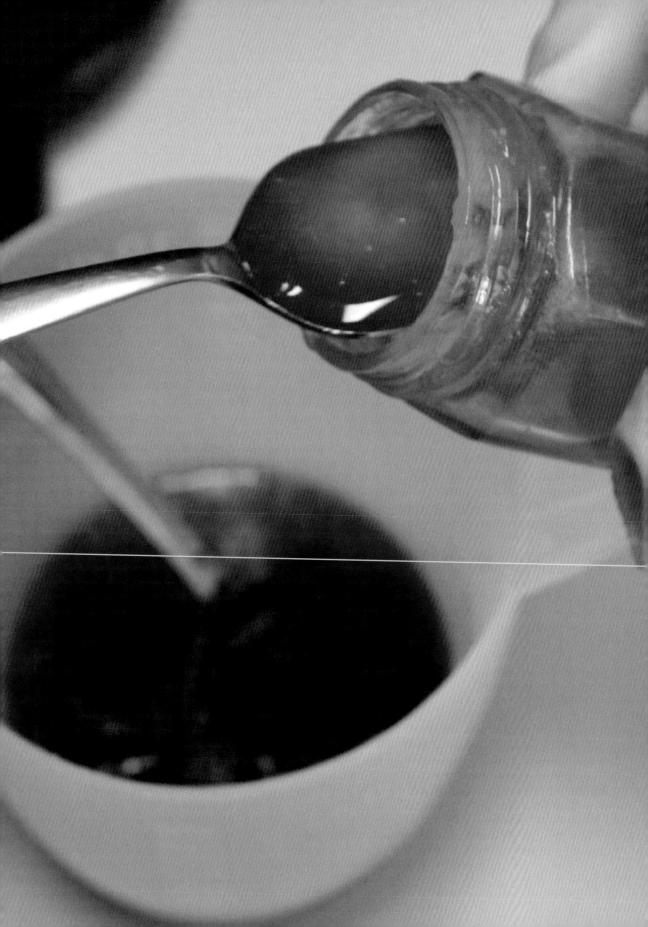

Honey bee bar

I've included both honey and beeswax in this soap. The beeswax will help to make the final result a hard bar but can also accelerate trace, so don't hang around once you have reached trace – just get the soap into the mould as soon as you can! I haven't included any additional aroma as the natural honey lye gives a subtle sweet aroma.

You will also need a sheet of bubble wrap to place on top of the soap during the first 24 hours.

LYE SOLUTION
168 g water • 60 g sodium hydroxide • 30 g honey

SOAP OILS AND BUTTERS
100 g coconut oil • 265 g olive oil • 35 g beeswax • 50 g shea butter

METHOD
Line your mould if necessary and place to one side.

Wearing safety equipment (page 10), make up your lye solution using the water and sodium hydroxide. Add the honey and stir again. The lye will go through various colours of orange to brown and start to smell of treacle-like caramel. Set this safely aside somewhere out of the way.

Weigh the oils, beeswax and shea butter and put them into a saucepan. Place the pan over a low heat until the butter has melted.

Wearing your safety goggles and gloves and paying careful attention to the safe handling of the honey lye (page 9), pour the honey lye into the melted butter, beeswax and oils mixture.

Stir briefly with a spoon to mix the oils and lye together. Blitz with a stick blender until you have reached trace.

Pour the soap mixture (or dollop it, if it has started to turn very thick) into your prepared mould.

Place a layer of bubble wrap onto the soap with the protruding bubbles facing down. Smooth this onto the soap. Cover the mould with a lid, chopping board a or piece of cardboard and then cover with one layer of towel and leave for 24 hours.

Remove the soap from the mould when it is hard enough. Carefully peel back the bubble wrap and discard it. The bubble wrap indents should give the soap a similar appearance to honeycomb.

*Covering your honey soap
with a layer of bubble wrap
gives a honeycomb effect*

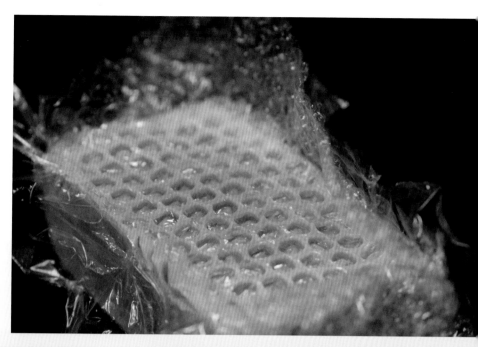

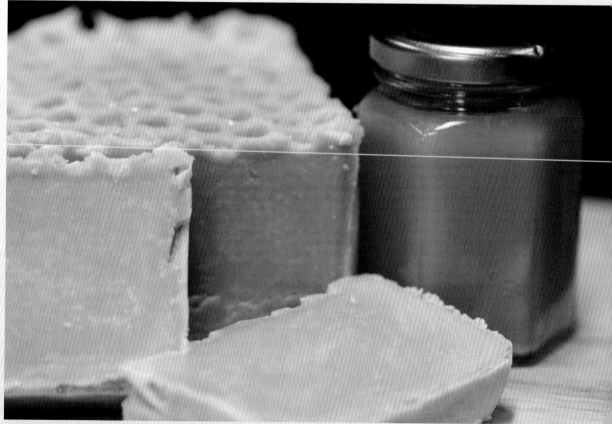

Honey bee bars

Honey and oats soap

My son always used to call this 'flapjack soap' since it not only looked like an oaty bar but had the aroma of something you might like to eat. But no matter how tempted you are, don't eat it – it will taste vile! I know, my son told me.

As the oats will make an exfoliating bar, you could choose to add them to half the soap so that the other half can remain smooth and perfect for those areas where you don't need to exfoliate! This is the method described in this recipe.

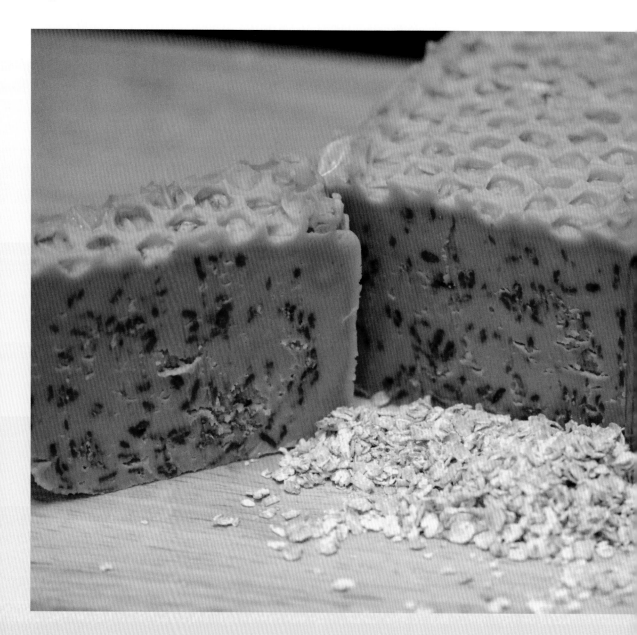

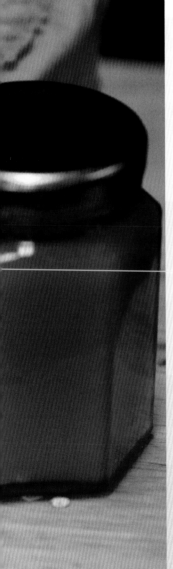

LYE SOLUTION
168 g water • 60 g sodium hydroxide • 30 g honey

SOAP OILS
50 g coconut oil • 50 g wheatgerm oil • 100 g sweet almond oil
100 g olive oil • 100 g rice bran oil • 50 g palm oil

ADDITION
30 g oats

METHOD
Make and bring the soap mixture to trace as for the Honey bee bar (page 120).

Pour half the soap mixture into a jug and set aside. Add the oats to the remaining soap in the saucepan and stir well. Pour the oaty soap mixture into the mould.

Now pour the remaining soap mixture in the jug onto the oaty layer being careful not to dislodge the oaty layer too much.

Cover the mould with a lid, chopping board or a piece of cardboard and cover with a layer of towel and leave for 24 hours.

Remove the soap from the mould when it is hard enough and slice into bars.

*Melt-and-pour soap with
added honey and oats*

Milk and honey

This is one of my favourite soaps. The inclusion of the argan oil makes it my guilty pleasure, but oh, my skin feels clean, soft and silky after showering! We have our own bees so I use our own honey. I've tried to persuade my husband to let me have a goat too, but he's drawn the line at that one so I had to buy in my goats' milk.

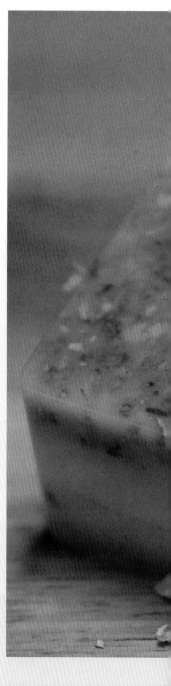

Lye solution
68 g water • 61 g sodium hydroxide • 30 g honey • 100 g frozen goats' milk

Soap oils
100 g castor oil • 150 g olive oil • 100 g wheatgerm oil
100 g coconut oil

Soap scent
12 g vanilla bourbon fragrance oil

Addition
15 g argan oil

Method
Stand your lye jug in the sink. Make up the lye as usual with the water, sodium hydroxide and honey. Add the frozen goats' milk and stir until the sodium hydroxide has dissolved.

Place the oils in a saucepan and heat until melted. Remove from the heat and fetch the lye.

Carefully pour the lye into the soap mixture and stir gently. Then blitz with a handheld blender until you have reached a light trace.

Add the vanilla bourbon fragrance oil and argan oil and stir until thoroughly incorporated into the soap mixture.

Cover the soap mould with a piece of cardboard or lid and place in the fridge for 24 hours. Remove from the fridge but leave in the mould until the soap is hard enough to remove easily. Cut into slices but do not use the soap until it is at least six weeks old.

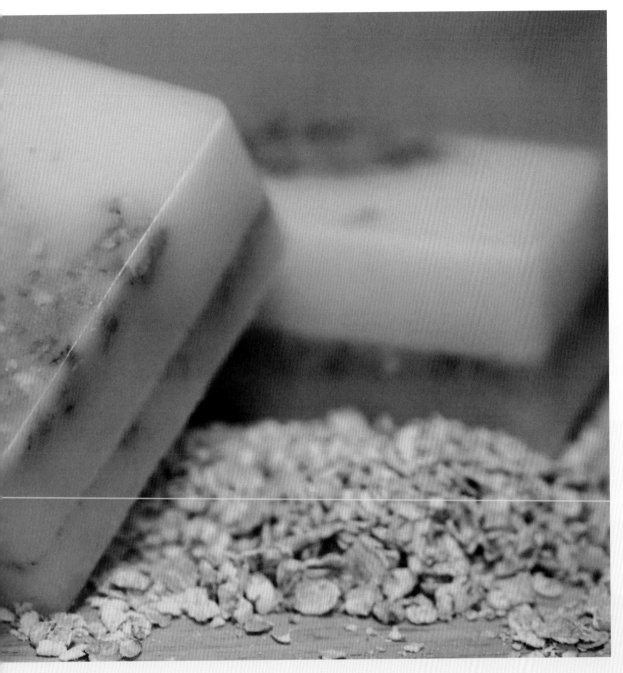

Milk and honey soap

Adding salt to your soaps

Adding salt to soap will make the bar harder. Whilst salt may be added to the lye solution, it can also be added to the traced soap mixture or scattered on top of the soap, making it an exfoliating bar. Most salt types can be used, including sea salt, table salt, Epsom salts and Himalayan salts. I haven't had much success using Dead Sea salt as I found it made the soap overly crumbly in parts.

Pink and gold salt bars

Here, I have used Himalayan pink salt to add colour as well as texture. The salt is added once the soap has been poured into the moulds and will sit on top of the soap, making this an exfoliating bar.

LYE SOLUTION
168 g water • 68 g sodium hydroxide

SOAP OILS AND BUTTERS
100 g coconut oil • 50 g palm oil • 250 g olive oil • 50 g shea butter

SOAP SCENT
12 g frankincense essential oil

COLOUR
1 g gold mica

ADDITION
50 g Himalayan salt

METHOD

Make up your lye as usual with the water and sodium hydroxide (page 11). Leave to one side whilst you prepare the oils and butter.

Place the oils and butter in a saucepan and heat until everything has melted. Remove from the heat and carefully add the lye.

Bring the soap to a light trace then add the frankincense essential oil.

Remove one third of the soap mixture and place it in a separate jug. Add the gold mica to this and stir well.

Pour half the uncoloured soap mixture into your prepared mould. Carefully pour the gold mica layer on top of the uncoloured layer. Pour the remaining uncoloured soap mixture on top of the gold mica layer. Sprinkle the Himalayan salt on top of the soap mixture.

Cover the soap mould with a piece of cardboard or lid and insulate with towels or blankets (page 38).

Remove the towels and blankets after 24 hours. Once the soap is hard, cut it into slices, sprinkling any wayward salt back onto the soap bars. The soap is ready to use in four weeks.

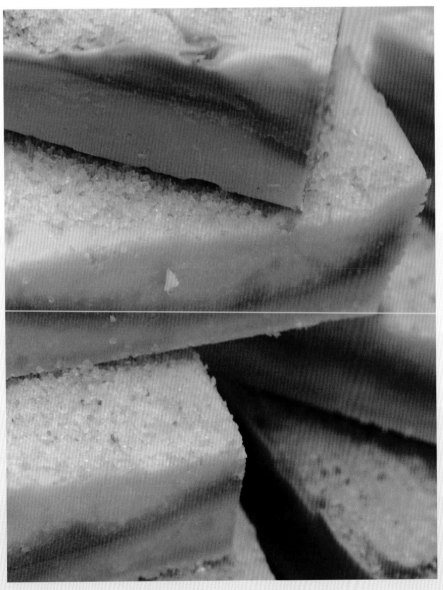

Pink and gold salt bars

Adding silk to your soaps

The addition of silk to your soaps will make the soap creamy, silky and absolutely gorgeous! Silk can be found in fibre, liquid or powder format, but easily the most cost-effective form is the silk fibres.

Whatever form of silk you choose to use, add it to the lye. The powder and liquid silks dissolve into the lye straightaway, but silk fibres take a while to dissolve. I often make this lye the day before I need it, allowing plenty of time for the silk fibres to disperse.

Silky skin treat

The inclusion of silk and argan oil makes this one very special soap. Tussah silk fibres are humanely harvested from the cocoons of wild silk moths. They add a lovely silk feel to your soap and to your skin after using it.

LYE SOLUTION
168 g water • 62 g sodium hydroxide • 2 g tussah silk fibres

SOAP OILS AND BUTTERS
50 g argan oil • 50 g castor oil • 100 g coconut oil
100 g olive oil • 50 g palm oil • 100 g shea butter

SOAP SCENT
12 g coriander essential oil

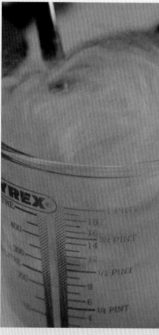

METHOD
Make up your lye with the water and sodium hydroxide as usual (page 11). Add the silk fibres and leave to dissolve (this may take several hours).

Place the oils and butter in a saucepan and heat until everything has melted. Remove from the heat and carefully add the silky lye.

Bring the soap to a light trace then add the coriander essential oil.

Pour the soap into your mould, cover with a piece of cardboard or a lid and insulate (page 38) with towels or blankets.

Remove from the towels and blankets after 24 hours and leave the soap to cure at room temperature for four weeks.

Adding tussah silk fibres to the lye

Superfatting your soap

The bar soaps you make are likely to be creamy, moisturising and wonderfully rich in lather, making them a treat to use. It is possible to make them even creamier and more moisturising, though by adding excess oils to the soap mixture. This procedure is called superfatting your soap.

It is important not to add too much excess oil as this will have an impact on the lathering capabilities of your soap. You shouldn't use oils to superfat liquid soaps as the mixture will separate out (see Chapter Two). Use a fatty dispersant instead, such as sulphonated castor oil or polysorbate.

HOW TO SUPERFAT YOUR SOAPS

Superfatting your soaps can be done in one of two ways. The first method is to let the soap saponification calculators do the hard work for you, the second method is to do the very easy maths yourself. Whilst you might be breathing a sigh of relief and thinking that letting the calculator do the work for you is the easiest way to do this, it isn't necessarily the best option for those of us who like to have control over the superfatting oil. This is because the soap calculator will reduce the amount of sodium hydroxide required rather than increase the amount of oil.

This means that the unsaponified, excess oils 'floating around invisibly' in your soaps will be a mixture of your base oils rather than one particular, carefully selected oil.

If your soap recipe uses coconut oil, olive oil, palm oil and sweet almond oil and you superfat using the soap calculator method, what happens is that the calculation reduces the quantity of sodium hydroxide so not all the oils are converted into soap, only 95 per cent of them are. This is perfectly acceptable and your soap will be noticeably creamier and even more moisturising than if you haven't superfatted.

However, if you superfat using the manual calculation method, you can then choose to add a special extra oil to your soap at the trace stage and it is this oil that will float around invisibly. Argan, jojoba and other luxury and expensive oils are good examples of oils that you would want to superfat with in this way as this guarantees that it is these oils that are going to be the additional emollient oils in your soap.

MANUALLY CALCULATING HOW MUCH OIL TO SUPERFAT WITH

You can successfully superfat with an additional 5 per cent of the other soap oils you are using. Any more than that and your soap becomes greasy and will not produce much lather.

The recipes in this book use 450 g oils so the maximum amount you would consider adding as a superfatting oil is 22.5 g.

This is calculated by working out the value of 1 per cent and then multiplying that value by five to get 5 per cent. The calculation for our soaps is therefore as follows:

450g/100 = 4.5 g

Therefore 4.5 g is 1 per cent of our soap recipe. Hence: 4.5 g x 5 = 22.5 g

Therefore 22.5 g is the maximum additional oil we can include in our soap as a superfatting oil.

It is acceptable to include less than 22.5 g superfatting oil but do not add more. This oil is added at light trace and I always add it at the same time as I add my fragrance or essential oils.

Examples of recipes where I have successfully superfatted in this way include Rosy hue soap and the Milk and honey soap recipes (pages 55 and 124–25).

USING THE SOAP CALCULATOR TO CALCULATE SUPERFATTING

All the soap calculators on the internet are formatted differently so you may need to hunt around your preferred calculator page to find the superfatting field. Once you find the relevant area you will need to enter your required superfatting percentage into the field and it is likely that this field will accept values from 0 through to 5. If you want to superfat at the full 5 per cent then enter '5' into this field. If you do not wish to superfat at all, or wish to perform the calculation yourself then enter '0' in this field.

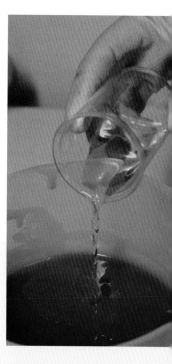

Adding 5 per cent excess oil to superfat the soap mixture

If you plan to calculate the superfatting oil yourself using the manual method you must make sure that the value in the soap calculator field is set to '0' otherwise you will over-superfat and your soap will definitely be too greasy.

The soap calculation method will not increase the oils, but will decrease the amount of sodium hydroxide required. The result is the same in that there will be excess oils in your soap.

Discounting the water in your soap

Reducing the amount of water in your soap is not technically a superfatting method, but I thought it best to include it in this section. If you refer back to the section on calculating how much water to use in your soap (page 23), you will see that most soap recipes calculate the amount of water to use as being approximately 37.5 per cent of the weight of oils.

Most of the recipes in this book use 450 g oils and therefore use approximately 168 g water (or water substitute), which is 37.5 per cent of the weight of the oils. In fact, the amount of water you use in your soaps can vary enormously. Some soap recipes use less, others more and one soap calculator suggests a range of 112 g–169 g for our 450 g oil recipe. So does it really matter? The answer is yes and no! Yes, in that the 37.5 per cent of the oils value is the ideal amount required to dissolve the lye to enable it to react with the oils, converting them into the fatty acids and glycerols required to create a beautiful block of soap, but also no, because you can put in less water if you wish and still convert the oils into soap. There is, however, a limit to how little water you can use, since the water is needed to dissolve the lye. If you don't have enough, the lye can't dissolve and there may be sections of undissolved sodium hydroxide in your soap.

The benefit of adding less water is that your soap will reach a thick trace fairly quickly. This is very useful if you wish to layer it, as the individual layers are less likely to run into each other. Discounting the water will also harden the soap up faster, in turn making the curing time quicker.

The disadvantages of adding less water are that the soap is more prone to seizing and it may harden up before you have time to pour it neatly into the mould. Please be aware that your lye solution will be more concentrated and therefore stronger than usual since you have used less water. Always wear your safety protective gear (page 10) when handling lye, regardless of the strength of the solution.

Hot process soaps should not be water-discounted as they tend to err on the side of dry. In fact, I sometimes add a little more hot water to my soaps during their cooking phase to make up for any water lost through evaporation.

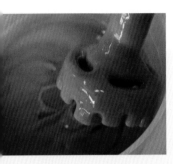

This soap has traced to a thicker mixture due to reducing the volume of water in the lye

HOW TO DISCOUNT THE WATER IN YOUR SOAP

Firstly please don't discount the water if you are using milks or purées in your soap. Also, don't rush into this, for it is a method used by experienced soap makers and it is wise to only try it once you feel comfortable making soap with the regular amount of liquid.

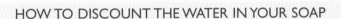

The lowest amount of water I suggest you go to is 25 per cent of the weight of the oils. This is calculated by dividing the weight of the oils by 100 and then multiplying it by 25. For our batches of soap made with 450 g oil, the calculation would look as follows: 450g/100 x 37.5 = 168 g. Therefore 168 g is the amount of water needed at 37 per cent.

The lowest percentage I recommend is 25 per cent. To calculate how much water this equates to, divide 450 g by 100 but this time multiply the result by 25. The formula would look like this: 450 g/100 x 25 = 112.5 g. Therefore 112.5 g is the amount of water needed at 25 per cent.

The amount of water required for a 450 g oil batch would therefore range from 112.5 g to 168 g. You can experiment by reducing the water, but start with a little reduction rather than reducing it to the full 25 per cent so that you learn how water discounts change the behaviour of your soap.

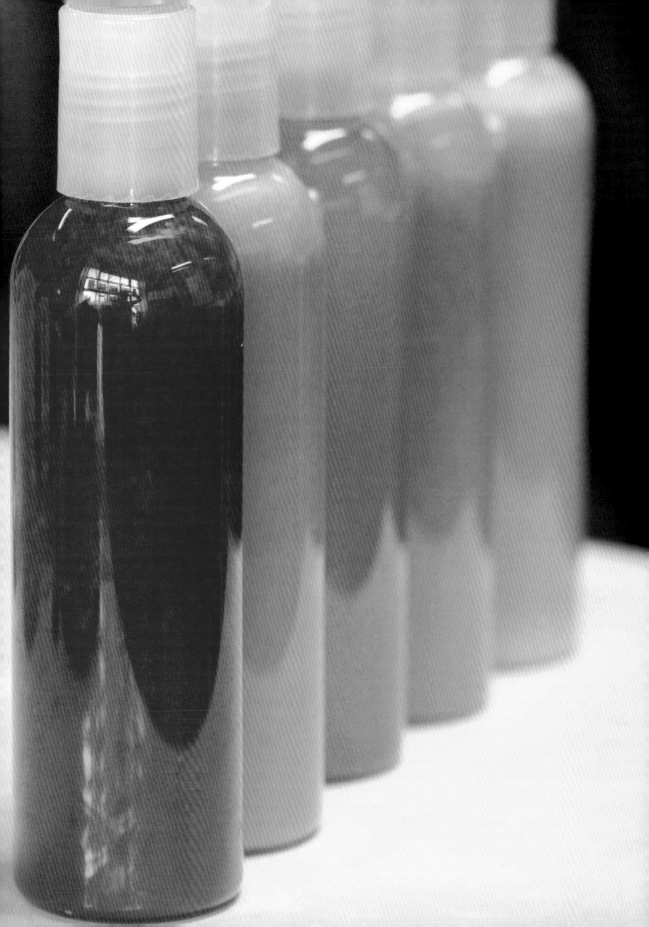

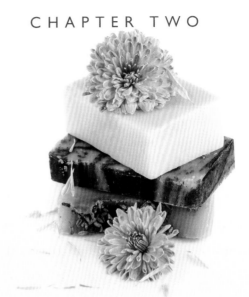

CHAPTER TWO

Making liquid soap

Liquid soap has gained in popularity over the last decade and, bottle for bar, it now outsells other types of soap.

The process of making liquid soap is more time consuming than making hard bars of soap, but can be made time-economical since making a large quantity requires little more effort than making a few bottles. Liquid soap is a very versatile product and can be modified easily to become hand soap, body wash, bubble bath and so on, by adding a selection of appropriate additional ingredients. Whilst it can take a while for your liquid soap to be 'cooked', it is certainly worth the wait. Alas liquid soap, in my opinion, will never look as beautiful and wholesome as hard bars of soap and much of the visual appeal of the final product will be down to the packaging, not just the product itself.

The liquid soap in this section is made from scratch using potassium hydroxide. It is also possible to make liquid soap products from surfactants – please refer to the chapter on using surfactants if you prefer that method of soap making (page 197). Your finished liquid soap will not contain any potassium hydroxide as it will have been transformed, with the oils and fats, into lovely liquid soap. Without the potassium hydroxide, the oils and water would separate, leaving you with a greasy, inexplicable, non-foaming mess!

Equipment needed for making liquid soap

A range of handmade liquid soaps

Very little specialist equipment is required to make liquid soap. The method I have included in this book requires the use of a slow cooker (crock-pot). It is perfectly feasible to make liquid soap in a saucepan, but there is a greater risk of the soap paste burning unless you are prepared to stir it frequently to ensure the soap is cooked evenly.

USING A DOUBLE BOILER FOR LIQUID SOAP

Using a double boiler will help reduce the chances of the soap burning. To make a double boiler, you will need a very large saucepan and another saucepan that fits snuggly inside the big saucepan. Add water to the outer big saucepan and heat this up. Insert the smaller saucepan into the big saucepan making sure that no water from the outer pan gets into the smaller pan. All your cooking is then carried out in the smaller saucepan.

Both pans will need a lid and you will need to check the water levels in the bigger pan frequently to make sure it hasn't boiled dry.

USING A SLOW COOKER (CROCK-POT) FOR LIQUID SOAP

If you don't already own a slow cooker that you are willing to dedicate to your soap making, may I suggest that when making a purchase you choose a large one that has at least two heat settings. By large, I mean that you should purchase one with the capacity to hold at least 5 litres, since once you start using the soap and giving it to friends and family, you'll find that big batches become the norm and you will be frustrated if your slow cooker can't manage bulk making.

Jugs and bowls
You will need an assortment of jugs and bowls. These can be used when weighing the water and potassium hydroxide, mixing the lye and weighing the diluted liquid soap. Heatproof glass or plastic jugs that can hold up to 2 litres are suitable.

Spoons and spatulas
You will need large stainless steel spoons for mixing the lye, soap paste and diluted liquid soap. Invest in a flexible spatula so that you can scrape the soapy residue from the sides of your slow cooker pot or saucepan.

Scales
You will need a set of accurate digital scales for measuring ingredients.

Handheld stick blender
This is required to bring your oils and lye mixture to the thick trace stage.

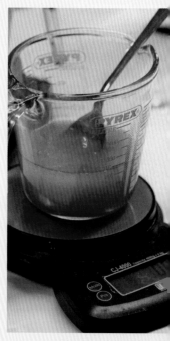

Digital scales help you to be more accurate when weighing out your ingredients

Protective clothing

As previously, you will need safety glasses, gloves, an apron and possibly a protective face mask. If you have long hair, you will need to tie it back.

Lidded containers or ziplock bags

Use these to store excess soap paste. The soap paste will remain fresh for at least 18 months if stored in an airtight container.

Bottles

You will need an assortment of bottles to put your finished product in.

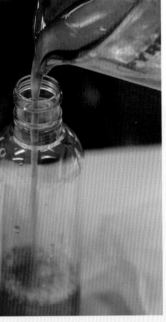

Pouring liquid soap into a bottle

Safety advice for handling liquid soap ingredients

Liquid soap is made in a similar way to hot process hard bars of soap. The same safety rules apply so please read the lye safety section (pages 9 and 10) before starting to make liquid soaps.

Authentic, natural hard bar and liquid soap is made from the chemical reaction of lye combined with fats. The lye is made from water (or water combined with other liquids) and an alkali. For hard bars of soap, the alkali is sodium hydroxide; for liquid soaps, the alkali is potassium hydroxide.

Please see the section on handling lye safely for full instructions on how to make up your lye solution (pages 9–12).

LIQUID SOAP INGREDIENTS

Liquid soap is a mixture of oils and/or butters and potassium lye. There are only a few ingredients that you absolutely need to include in your recipes to achieve outstanding results. These comprise potassium hydroxide, water and oils or butters such as coconut oil, olive oil, almond oil, shea butter and such like.

Other soap making ingredients can be included, such as fragrances, colours, superfatting ingredients and specialist additives, depending on what liquid soap product you are making.

LIQUID SOAP INGREDIENTS – WATERS

During your liquid soap making you will add water at two different stages. The first stage is making up the lye solution and for this you can use regular tap water if you wish. If you live in an area that has very hard or soft tap water then you may want to consider deionised, distilled or spring water instead. The second stage of adding water is when you dilute your thick soap paste. Again, you can use tap water but we prefer to use spring or distilled water. You can substitute all or part of the dilution water with specialist waters such as floral waters, including rose or lavender water, or aloe vera. See the individual recipes for ideas and suggestions.

LIQUID SOAP INGREDIENTS – OILS AND BUTTERS

Any oil or butter that you would consider using in handmade cosmetic products can be used to make liquid soap. Each oil or butter brings different properties to the liquid soap and will have an impact on the skin feel, lathering ability and the appearance and colour of the soap itself.

Oils and butters are made up of different fatty acids that affect the characteristic and quality of your liquid soap. 'Hard' oils, such as coconut and palm kernel oils or shea butter, tend to have high stearic fatty acid content since it is the occurrence of stearic acid that keeps these oils solid at ambient temperatures. These oils may also contain other fatty acids such as palmitic and lauric acids, all of which will have an impact on your final liquid soap product.

'Soft' oils, such as almond, olive, peach kernel and castor, are usually liquid at ambient temperatures. They too may contain stearic, palmitic and lauric fatty acids but in much smaller quantities than their more solid, oily counterparts. Soft oils are more likely to contain larger proportions of oleic, linoleic and linolenic fatty acids. The fatty acid content will help to determine how the liquid soap feels on your skin, as well as how clear, foaming, moisturising and viscous it is.

FATTY ACID CONTENT OF OILS

Use the following chart to help you decide which oils and butters you should use in your liquid soap product. For example, if you wish to have a richly moisturising liquid soap that has a long-lasting lather, then oils with palmitic and ricinoleic acids will be beneficial. Oils rich in these fatty acids include castor oil (ricinoleic)

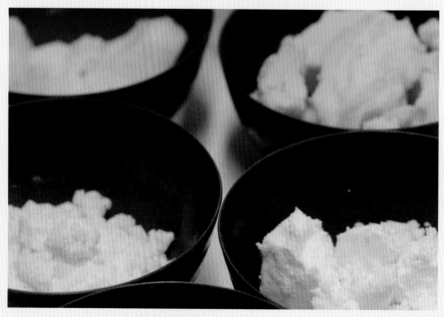

Basic ingredients required for liquid soap making

and cocoa butter, olive, palm, peach kernel, rice bran, rosehip and wheatgerm oils. These oils will not necessarily create a clear liquid soap. If you want a mostly clear soap, choose oils that have water-soluble fatty acids such as coconut or palm (lauric and myristic acids) and avocado (myristic acid). However, these fatty acids can be a little drying on the skin, so you would also need to include oils that contain moisturising fatty acids such as linoleic acid (which may be prone to rancidity) or oleic acid (which doesn't lather particularly well).

Fatty acid	Found in these oils	Characteristic in liquid soap
Lauric acid	Coconut, palm kernel	Antibacterial, antifungal properties Helps to create a quick, fluffy, foamy lather Water-soluble so helps produce a clear soap High lauric acid content can cause skin dryness
Linoleic acid	Borage, evening primrose, flaxseed, grape-seed, hemp, rosehip, safflower, sesame seed, sunflower, walnut, wheatgerm	Fabulous silky skin moisturisation and conditioning properties Anti-inflammatory properties Oils high in linoleic acid tend to have a shorter freshness and are prone to rancidity
Linolenic acid	Borage, evening primrose, hemp seed, flax seed, kukui nut	Skin moisturising Mild and therefore very suitable for sensitive skin types
Myristic acid	Avocado, coconut, palm kernel	Creates a fluffy lather Good cleansing properties May cause skin dryness Water-soluble so helps produce a clear soap Contributes to soap viscosity
Oleic acid	Almond, apricot kernel, avocado, hazelnut, olive, peach kernel, shea butter	Richly moisturising and conditioning Good skin feel Little lathering ability
Palmitic acid	Cocoa butter, olive, palm, peach kernel, rice bran, rosehip, wheatgerm	Produces long-lasting, stable lather Good skin moisturising ability Can make soap cloudy
Ricinoleic acid	Castor	Rich, stable, fluffy lather Great skin moisturisation About 80–90 per cent of castor oil is made up of ricinoleic fatty acid so it is worthy of a special mention. You don't need much castor oil to make a difference in the lathering and moisturising capabilities of your liquid soap
Stearic acid	Cocoa butter, coconut, jojoba, palm, shea butter	Rich, stable lather Improves viscosity of soap Can make soap cloudy

LIQUID SOAP INGREDIENTS – ADDITIONS

There are many ingredients that can be added to your liquid soap product to enhance the way it feels on your skin, how it smells, the colour, how long it lasts, to add viscosity and so on. Since liquid soap is a rinse-off product, it should be noted that the effects of ingredients included to treat the skin in any way are unlikely to be totally successful, given that the liquid soap product is only on your skin for a short time before being washed off. Active ingredients of this nature will therefore be more effective if included in a leave-on product.

Use this chart to decide what additions you can add to your liquid soap product to change its characteristics.

Ingredient	Function	Comments
Essential or fragrance oil	Adds an aroma	Essential oils will also bring active properties to your liquid soap, but since the soap is in contact with the skin for a very short time before it is rinsed away, we consider essential oils to be added for their wonderful aroma only. Essential and fragrance oils should be added at a maximum of 2 per cent Some essential oils contain sensitisers and should be kept to less than 1 per cent. Oils in this category include tea tree, clove, ginger and cinnamon. If in doubt, please seek advice from a qualified toxicologist or aromatherapist Some essential and fragrance oils may cause your liquid soap product to become cloudy even if you carefully select oils that help give clarity to your soap Add to the diluted soap
Glycerine	Adds glide and improves lather	Glycerine will improve the lathering capability of your liquid soap Add up to 50 per cent to make a bubble bath Glycerine can be added to the soap paste or to the diluted soap
Cyclomethicone	Adds a silky feel	Add up to 5 per cent to the diluted soap
Oat or silk protein	Adds a silky feel (silk) and skin softness (oat)	Add up to 5 per cent to diluted soap Silk protein is available in both powder and liquid form Dissolve powdered silk protein in a little water before adding it to the diluted soap
Polyquaternium-7	Anti-static, skin conditioning	Any of the amphoteric 'quats' (a cosmetic ingredient that conditions skin and hair) will help to reduce static, as well as offering skin-conditioning properties Add between 0.5–1 per cent

D-panthenol	Soothing, healing, anti-inflammatory, protective	D-panthenol, also known as vitamin B5, can help dry, sensitive skin and gives your liquid soap a superior skin feel D-panthenol also helps add viscosity to liquid soap Add during the diluting phase at up to 5 per cent
Polysorbate, sulphonated castor oil, sucragel	Superfatting	These oils are water-soluble and will disperse in the diluted liquid soap. They are used to add an extra moisturising boost to your liquid soap, but need to be mixed well to ensure that they don't separate Add the superfatting ingredient at a rate of up to 5 per cent of your diluted soap
Gum	Thickener	Getting liquid soap to thicken can be quite a challenge. Most cosmetic gums can be used to create a gel that can then be added to change the viscosity of liquid soap. You can add the gum directly to your diluted liquid soap, but it will take a few hours to dissolve and thicken Gums such as xanthan, tara, guar, carrageenan, Arabic and cellulose can all be used. Each of these gums has slightly different thickening capabilities so you will need to experiment to find which one you prefer to work with. Start with 1 per cent and then work up or down from there
Salt	Thickener	Common table salt, sea salt and Dead Sea salt will all thicken your liquid soap but they may also turn the soap cloudy Do experiment as some essential or fragrance oils will cause the salt to split the liquid soap rather than thicken it
Colour	Adds colour	A drop or two of liquid colour will disperse very effectively in diluted liquid soap. A little goes a long way, so do use sparingly. Due to the natural colour of the oils, the liquid soap is likely to have a naturally golden colour. You will need to take this into account when adding a different colour to the liquid soap. If you add a drop of blue, it will mix with the gold and give you a greenish tint Water-soluble powder colours may be used too. Mix with a little water before adding them to your diluted liquid soap Mica can be used, but the slight alkali nature of the soap can fade some micas
Preservative	Extends shelf life	The lye will kill off any lurking microbes during the paste making stage. Since this then gets diluted with additional water, the shelf life is shortened Natural liquid soap will have a shelf life of about six months Adding preservative extends the shelf life to 18 months (depending on the preservative and percentage you use)

How to make liquid soap

Liquid soap will take up to eight hours from start to finish although this depends on the oils you use, the volume of soap you are making and how much time you are prepared to dedicate to stirring and fussing over your soap. There are various time and labour saving techniques which you can adopt as you develop your soap making. Although you can make liquid soap in a large saucepan, there is more risk of it burning unless it is stirred regularly. I recommend you use a slow cooker (crock-pot) as you need attend to it only occasionally.

Before embarking on your liquid soap making, read through the lye handling instructions (pages 9 and 10) and the liquid soap recipe you are going to follow and make sure you have everything to hand before you start.

MAKING LIQUID SOAP

Step 1

Weigh the oils and/or butters and place them in the slow cooker (crock-pot). Turn on the slow cooker (stock-pot) to melt them.

Step 2

Wearing safety clothing (page 10), make your lye by adding the carefully measured out potassium hydroxide to the weighed water in a well-ventilated room. Stir until the potassium hydroxide has dissolved. Make sure that you adhere to all the safety instructions as the lye will be very caustic and extremely hot at this stage, and will be releasing fumes that may make you cough.

Step 3

Turn your slow cooker to low, pour the lye over the melted oils and stir well using a spoon.

Once you have mixed the oils and lye, use a stick blender to mix further until you have reached a light trace (where the soap mixture has thickened slightly and looks more like a batter than an oily liquid). As you lift the stick blender out of the mixture, drizzle the dripping soap batter on top of the soap mixture in the pot. It should sit momentarily on top of the batter before merging into the mix. The mixture may try to separate and curdle, please don't worry: this is normal. Just keep blending to bring the mixture together again.

If you are used to making cold or hot process soap you will find that it takes longer for the liquid soap oils and lye to reach light trace. To save burning out your stick blender, blend for a few minutes at a time, let the mixture (and blender) rest for a few minutes and then blend again.

Once you have reached light trace, you will need to mix with the stick blender until you have reached a heavy trace. Be prepared for this to take at least half an hour of intermittent blending and resting, although the exact

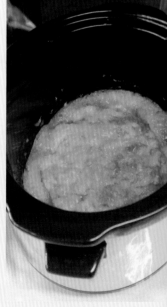

Liquid soap cooking

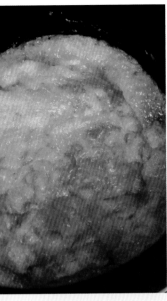

timings depend on the type of oils, temperature and volume of the mixture, and the power of your stick blender. You needn't blend for the full time – in fact, please don't or you will definitely burn out the blender's motor! Blend on and off until thick trace has been reached.

Step 4

Place the lid on the slow cooker and cook for two hours or so, stirring the soap mixture every 20–30 minutes. Use a spatula to scrape down any of the soap mixture that rises up the sides of the slow cooker pot.

Step 5

When the liquid soap is 'cooked' and ready it will be smooth and glossy and similar to Vaseline in appearance although not in colour. It will probably be a golden to amber colour, but this depends on the oils that you have used. Make sure that you have thoroughly mixed in all the liquid soap mixture – right down to the parts lurking at the bottom of the pot and the soap residue that has climbed up the sides of it.

Step 5: Liquid soap reaching the glossy stage

The cooking of your liquid soap will take up to three hours depending on the size of the batch and the type of oils you have used.

Liquid soap cooked to a paste

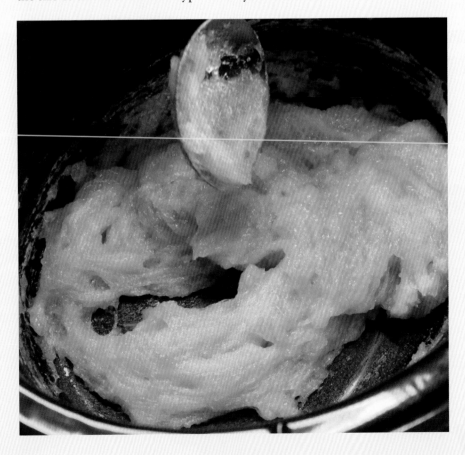

Step 6

If you are unsure whether your liquid soap is cooked and ready, place a heaped teaspoon (approximately 10 g) of liquid soap mixture in 25 g of very hot spring water and stir until it has mostly dissolved. If the water is very cloudy, the liquid soap needs more cooking but if it is only a little cloudy or is mostly clear, the soap is ready for diluting.

The cooked soap mixture is now referred to as the 'soap paste'. Before it can be used on the body, it will need diluting.

Step 7

Diluting your liquid soap paste takes time, patience and a bit of strength to stir the thick paste. Before going ahead, you have a decision to make. Do you want to make all of your paste into liquid soap at this point, or do you wish to save some paste to use at a later date? If you decide to save some paste, remove a portion of the paste and pop it into a pot (do not put the lid on the pot until the paste has completely cooled). The paste can also be stored in a polythene ziplock bag, but do not put it into the bag until it is cool.

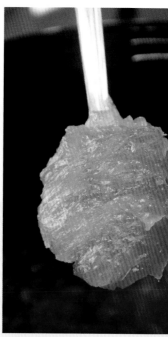

Liquid soap paste ready to dilute

The paste can be stored somewhere cool or in a fridge for at least 12 months. Whether you are diluting a fresh paste or diluting a paste that has been stored for a few months, the same rules for diluting soap paste apply. You will need to know the weight of the soap paste you wish to dilute. If your soap paste is still hot and in the slow cooker (crock-pot) then the easiest way of doing this is to weigh an empty jug and make a note of the weight. Carefully spoon the hot soap paste into the jug and weigh it again. Calculate the weight of the soap paste by taking the *full* jug weight and subtracting the *empty* jug weight – the result is the weight of the soap paste.

DILUTING YOUR SOAP PASTE

The amount of water you need to dilute your soap paste very much depends on the oils you used to make the soap paste. Water-soluble fatty acids such as lauric and myristic acid found in coconut or palm (lauric and myristic acids) and avocado (myristic acid) will require less water to dilute than a soap paste made with oils high in stearic or palmitic acid, such as shea butter or rice bran oil.

I always recommend starting with less water than you think you need since you can always add more later – if you add more water than you actually need, you will need to thicken your liquid soap and this is not so easy.

Start by adding equal weights of hot spring water to soap paste. Pour the hot spring water over the soap paste and give it a stir. When you stir you will simply be shifting the soap paste around in the water and not dissolving it, so please don't be surprised when nothing seems to change in the pot! Dissolving the soap paste takes time. I usually do this stage in the evening – I heat the water and paste up to not-quite-boiling temperature and then turn the slow

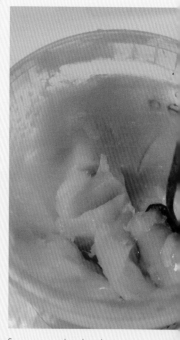

Soap paste that has been stored for a few months

cooker (crock-pot) off and go to bed. When I come down in the morning, my diluted liquid soap paste awaits me. Never be tempted to leave the slow cooker on overnight.

Step 8

Your soap paste will now be dissolved and you will have a pot full of unscented liquid soap. Depending on how much water you added, you may find much of the soap has dissolved but there is a thick skin on top of it. If this is the case, peel back the skin and carefully pour off the liquid soap into a jug.

The skin is undiluted soap paste, which can be dissolved by adding more water. Weigh the skin and add equal amounts of not-quite-boiling spring water. Bring the mixture to simmering point and then turn the heat off and leave it for a few hours.

Step 9

Test the pH value of your soap to make sure that it is mild enough to go on the skin. You are aiming for a pH value of around 6–9 (lower is better). Use pH papers, a pH meter (available from specialist online lab suppliers) or phenolphthalein to test the pH (overleaf).

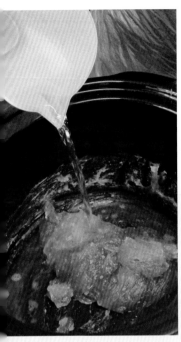

Diluting the soap paste

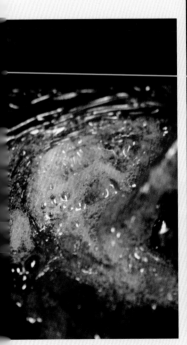

Diluted soap ready to colour, fragrance and bottle

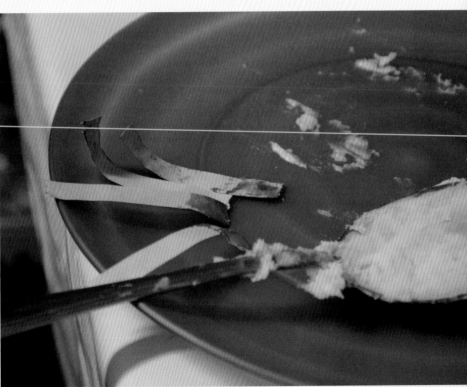

pH papers will go a shade of green when the soap is at the right level

HOW TO PERFORM A PHENOLPHTHALEIN TEST

For me, this is always a favourite test as it can produce the most beautiful fuchsia pink! However, pink isn't the colour you want on this occasion. You need the liquid soap to be clear to pale pink, which indicates a neutral or 'skin friendly' pH reading.

Dilute two drops of phenolphthalein in 250 ml water and stir well. Place a little of your soap mixture in a beaker and add 30 ml of the diluted phenolphthalein mixture. If it turns bright pink, the soap is a little too alkali; if clear or pale pink, your mixture is fine.

Alternatively, and in the absence of phenolphthalein, dip a pH paper (or meter) into the liquid soap to record its pH value. If the soap paper turns a shade of green, then the pH should be fine but if it is blue, the soap will need neutralising (see below).

NEUTRALISING YOUR LIQUID SOAP

If you need to bring the pH value down a little, add approximately 15–20 g of pH adjuster solution to your liquid soap mixture. To make a pH adjuster solution, mix 14 g citric acid with 56 g boiled water – this is at a ratio of one part citric acid to four parts water. Note that this may turn your soap a little cloudy and cause it to appear temporarily curdled. Stir and then leave the soap alone for a while to let it settle.

Step 10
You may wish to adjust the consistency of the diluted soap if it is too thin. Hot liquid soap mixture is naturally more viscous than a cold liquid soap mixture so you should wait until the mixture is cold before deciding whether or not to thicken. Any additional ingredient that you add, such as glycerine, oat protein, essential or fragrance oil, may have an impact on the viscosity so add these before thickening.

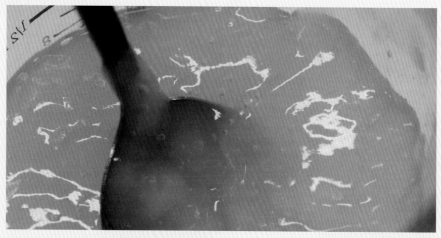

Step 11: Xanthan gel will thicken your liquid soaps

THICKENING YOUR LIQUID SOAP

If your liquid soap mixture is too runny, you can thicken it by using a little gum such as xanthan, tara, guar or gum Arabic.

Step 11

In a small bowl, combine half a teaspoon (2 g) gum to 50 g of the runny liquid soap base and stir well to ensure there are no lumps of gum remaining. Add a little of this mixture back into the runny liquid soap mixture and stir well. If necessary, add more of the gum mixture until you have the desired consistency.

Note that some gums are more robust than others and you may need to add a little more or a little less depending on which gum you use.

Depending on the oils you have used you may find it just as easy to thicken your mixture with salt. Add 2 per cent of the liquid soap weight in salt and stir well. Keep adding salt until you have reached the consistency you require. Do be warned that if you add too much salt, it can cause the mixture to thin up again so add the salt a little at a time, stirring between additions.

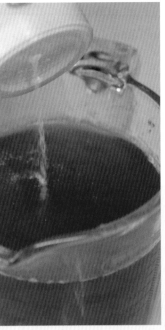

Step 11: Add table salt to thicken your liquid soaps

Step 12

Once you have achieved the correct pH value and the correct consistency, you can split the liquid soap into smaller quantities and add colour and up to 2 per cent essential or fragrance oils, plus any other additions such as d-panthenol, colour, glycerine or polysorbate before placing it in suitable containers.

Whilst the soap can be used straightaway, it may be a little harsh and have a slight 'bite'. Leaving your soap to rest for four weeks will help to make it milder. This resting period is called 'sequestering' and during this period the clarity of the soap may be improved, although this does depend on the oils, butters and fragrance you used.

Oils with a high palmitic and stearic acid content, such as shea butter, cocoa butter, jojoba and palm oil, will make your soap cloudy.

The shelf life of your liquid soap is six months. If you wish to keep it for longer, you can add a preservative.

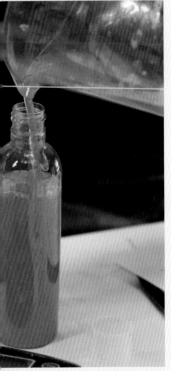

Step 12: Beautiful liquid soap!

RECIPES FOR LIQUID SOAP

These recipes take you as far as creating the soap paste although I have also included additions that you will need to include as part of the dilution stage. Eash recipe will yield approximately 1 litre liquid soap.

Refer to the more detailed stages earlier in this section (pages 140–145) for a full description of the steps necessary to make your liquid soap paste.

Make sure that you adhere to all the safety guidelines and wear protective clothing when making and handling your lye (page 10). There is no need to sterilise bottles but if you wish, you can swill them out with a diluted sterilisation solution such as those used for sterilising babies' bottles. Soap bottles are usually plastic, so they won't necessarily withstand using the heat method of sterilisation.

Gentle skin liquid soap

I have used oils rich in oleic acid here to help to moisturise and condition the skin. Since these aren't particularly good at creating a rich lather, I have added additional glycerine to boost the bubbles.

POTASSIUM LYE SOLUTION
56 g potassium hydroxide • 112 g water

LIQUID SOAP OILS
50 g shea butter • 150 g sweet almond oil • 100 g olive oil

LIQUID SOAP SCENT
2 per cent lavender essential oil

ADDITIONS
Up to 10 per cent glycerine • Blue liquid colouring

METHOD
Prepare the potassium lye solution (page 11).

Melt the shea butter, then remove the pan from the heat or turn off the slow cooker (crock-pot). Add the other liquid oils.

Slowly and carefully pour the lye solution into the saucepan or slow cooker. Stir the lye and oil mixture well to ensure that all the liquids are thoroughly combined. Then stir with a stick blender for two minutes before leaving the mixture to rest for two more minutes. After five minutes, stir again with a stick blender for two minutes then leave to rest.

Continue this process (stir for two minutes, rest for five minutes) until the liquid soap mixture reaches a heavy trace.

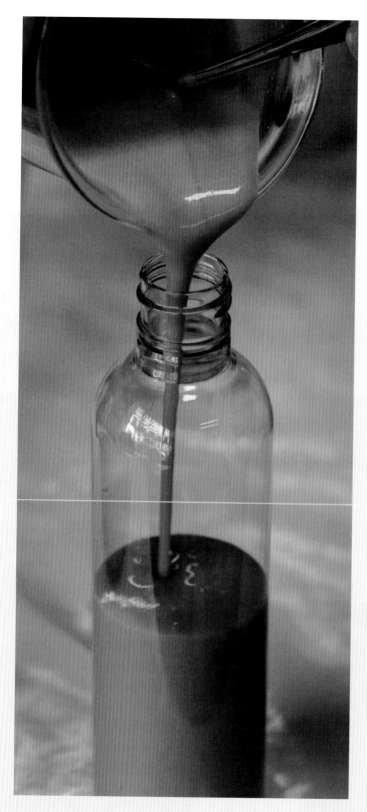

Put the mixture back on the heat, or turn the slow cooker on. Cook on a low heat setting, stirring every 10 minutes or so for the first hour. The liquid soap will migrate from a thick trace in appearance to a translucent apple sauce-type mixture. It will become thicker and more difficult to stir, but continue stirring every 20 minutes or so to ensure that all the noticeable oils are mixed into the liquid soap mixture. Cook the liquid soap until it is smooth and glossy, and similar to Vaseline in appearance.

If you wish to set aside some of the soap paste to use later (page 142), you can do that now. Weigh the remaining soap paste and add approximately an equal amount of hot water to it. Bring to a gentle boil and then turn the heat off and leave the soap to dissolve.

Once the liquid soap mixture has fully dissolved into the water, test the pH of the mixture (page 144) and adjust if necessary.

Thicken your liquid soap, if necessary using the gum or salt method, or a combination of the two (page 145).

Add lavender essential oil, glycerine and colouring; stir well before pouring into bottles.

Gentle skin liquid soap

Splash! body wash

A combination of myristic, oleic and palmitic acids in these oils produces a moisturising, cleansing soap with long-lasting bubbles. The ozonic aroma of the salty sea dog fragrance oil and the tingling freshness of the peppermint essential oil give this body wash a fresh, clean, energising aroma.

POTASSIUM LYE SOLUTION
44 g potassium hydroxide • 112 g water

LIQUID SOAP OILS
100 g rice bran oil • 100 g olive oil • 100 g coconut oil

LIQUID SOAP SCENT
1.5 per cent salty sea dog fragrance oil
0.5 per cent peppermint essential oil

ADDITIONS
Up to 5 per cent glycerine • Green liquid colouring

METHOD
Follow the instructions for the previous recipe, Gentle skin liquid soap, referring to the liquid soap making steps (pages 140–145) for more detail.

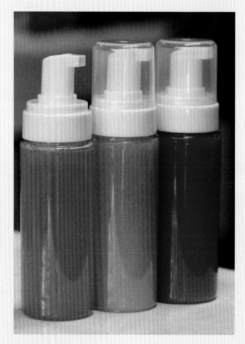

Foamer bottles are a useful alternative to thickening your liquid soaps

Beautiful body wash

An abundance of oils with high stearic, riconoleic and palmitic acids help to make this body wash very moisturising. I have suggested adding a little sulphonated castor oil with the dilution to give a superfatted, moisturising boost.

POTASSIUM LYE SOLUTION
50 g potassium hydroxide • 112 g water

LIQUID SOAP OILS
100 g castor oil • 50 g jojoba oil • 50 g rice bran oil
50 g wheatgerm oil • 50 g cocoa butter

LIQUID SOAP SCENT
2 per cent rose fragrance oil

ADDITIONS
5 per cent sulphonated castor oil • Pink liquid colouring

METHOD
Follow the instructions for the Gentle skin liquid soap recipe (page 146), referring to the liquid soap making steps (pages 140–145) for more detail. Add the sulphonated castor oil with the dilution water.

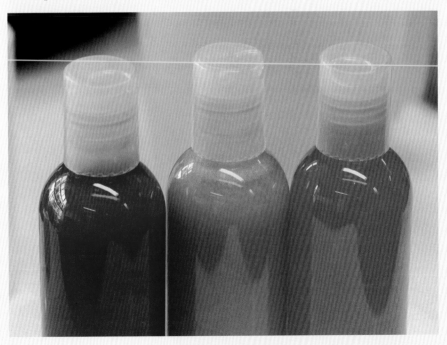

Beautiful body wash liquid soap

Sanity moisturising hand wash

With oils carefully selected for their moisturising capabilities and gentle foaming, this hand wash has an extra moisturising twist with the addition of polysorbate 80. Tea tree oil has natural antibacterial properties, as do oils high in lauric acid (coconut oil).

POTASSIUM LYE SOLUTION
59 g potassium hydroxide • 112 g water

LIQUID SOAP OILS
50 g cocoa butter • 50 g shea butter • 50 g avocado oil
50 g coconut oil • 100 g olive oil

LIQUID SOAP SCENT
1 per cent tea tree essential oil • 1 per cent lemon essential oil

ADDITION
5 per cent polysorbate 80

METHOD
Follow the instructions for the Gentle skin liquid soap recipe (page 146), referring to the liquid soap making steps (pages 140–145) for more detail. Add the polysorbate 80 with the dilution water.

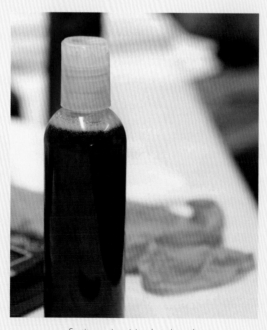

Sanity moisturising hand wash

Soft and gentle skin dew

Mild, gentle, skin softening and completely gorgeous, this liquid soap is suitable for sensitive skins, courtesy of the linolenic acid found in kukui nut oil and the d-panthenol. I've also included a little oat protein, which is very soothing.

POTASSIUM LYE SOLUTION
56 g potassium hydroxide • 112 g water

LIQUID SOAP OILS
50 g cocoa butter • 100 g sunflower oil • 100 g kukui nut oil
50 g castor oil

LIQUID SOAP SCENT
1 per cent amber fragrance oil • 0.5 per cent patchouli essential oil
0.5 per cent vanilla fragrance oil

ADDITIONS
5 per cent oat protein • 5 per cent d-panthenol

METHOD
Follow the instructions for the Gentle skin liquid soap recipe (page 146), referring to the liquid soap making steps (pages 140–145) for more detail. Add the oat protein and d-panthenol with the dilution water.

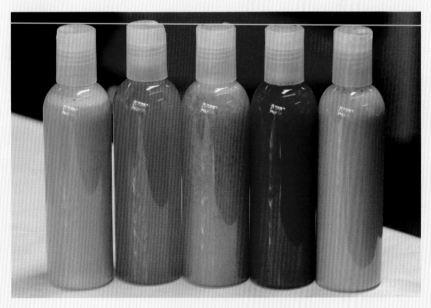

Liquid soaps ready for use

DESIGNING YOUR OWN LIQUID SOAP

There are plenty of soap calculators on the internet to help you to design your own liquid soap products.

Once you have decided which oils you would like to use to make your liquid soap, enter the quantity of the oils into a soap calculator and it will work out just how much potassium hydroxide and water you will need in order to make up the soap paste.

Always run your recipe through a liquid soap calculator such as the one found on the Plush Folly website www.plushfolly.com or one of the others listed here:

www.brambleberry.com/Pages/Lye-Calculator.aspx
www.summerbeemeadow.com/content/advanced-calculator-solid-cream-or-liquid-soaps
www.thesage.com/calcs/lyecalc2.php

CHAPTER THREE

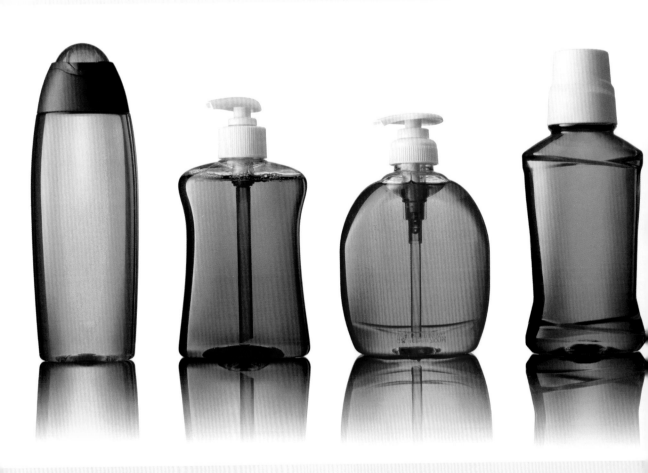

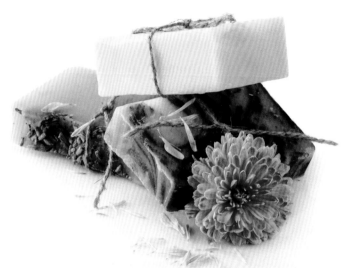

Making cream soap

Cream soap is mild, beautiful, ultra-moisturising and well worth the effort! It is much thicker and creamier than liquid soap, but softer than hard bars of soap. It's also a fun soap to use as it floats on the surface of the bath and feels very sensuous and luxurious when rubbed onto the skin.

Cream soap also makes a good shaving soap, especially if it contains rhassoul (a natural mineral clay from Morocco) or cosmetic clay to help give it 'slip'. Though it's not as well known as liquid or bar soaps, I thought it worth including a recipe or two for cream soap as it is so lovely to use.

The process is very similar to making liquid soap, but it is quicker and easier. Cream soap uses a combination of sodium and potassium hydroxides in the lye solution at a ratio of approximately five parts potassium hydroxide to one part sodium hydroxide.

Equipment needed for making cream soap

The equipment required to make cream soap is identical to the liquid soap equipment (page 133) but you will need a handheld electric whisk in addition to the stick blender. The stick blender is required to bring the mixture to a trace and the handheld whisk will make the final soap mixture froth up and become creamy.

In addition to the lye and the regular oils used in liquid and hard bars of soap, cream soap requires two other ingredients: glycerine and stearic acid.

Stearic acid is a fatty acid found in a number of oils, mainly coconut or other semi-solid oils. It is used to thicken cosmetics and to harden candles,

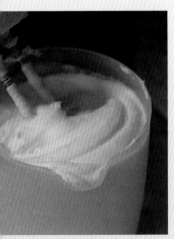

Whipped cream soap

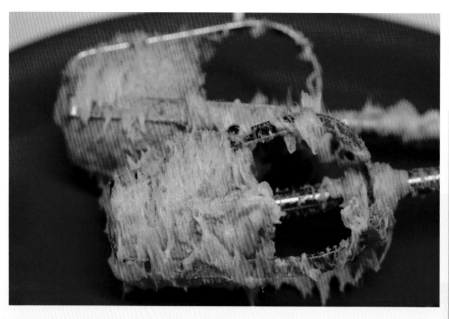

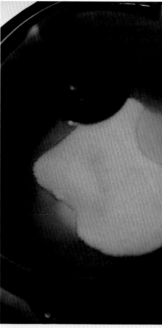

A handheld electric whisk will give added lightness to your soaps

allowing them to burn for longer. In addition, it gives the cream soap viscosity, texture and an almost opalescent shimmer. Stearic acid has a very high melting point so it takes a long time to melt.

Glycerine is a by-product of soap making, so your cream soap will be naturally glycerine-rich. Adding more glycerine will make it even more foamy, as well as soft, moisturising and gentle on your skin. The combination of lye, oils, stearic acid and glycerine results in a creamy, thick, semi-soft, moisturising, foaming soap.

Stearic acid will take the longest to melt of the oils and butters

---

Safety advice for handling cream soap ingredients

Cream soap is made in a similar way to liquid soap, but uses sodium hydroxide as well as potassium hydroxide. The same safety rules apply so please read the lye safety section (pages 9–12) before starting to make cream soaps.

How to make cream soap

Cream soap will take approximately three hours to make from start to finish although you will need to set time aside for it to rest and rot.

Step 1
Weigh and melt the oils and butters, including the stearic acid, in a slow cooker (crock-pot) or large saucepan. Please note that stearic acid takes much longer to melt than the other oils and butters (15 minutes as opposed to 5 minutes or so for oils and butters).

Step 2
Make your lye by adding the sodium and potassium hydroxides to water and stir until the hydroxides have dissolved (both can be added to the same water). Be sure to adhere to all the safety instructions as the lye will be very caustic at this stage and will be releasing fumes that may make you cough.

Step 3
Remove the melted oils, butters and stearic acid from the heat and add glycerine to the mixture.

Step 4
Add the lye to the melted oils mixture and stir using a stick blender. The mixture will immediately go lumpy and gloopy and look very odd – it will look as though the stearic acid has separated from the oils but don't worry, this is perfect natural. Blitzing with the handheld stick blender or stirring briskly with a stainless steel or silicone spoon will bring it back into the oils mixture.

Keep stirring on and off until the mixture is smooth and is a very, very thick plastic-looking paste. You may find that your stick blender becomes very hot so alternate between stirring with a spoon and stick blending, resting for a few minutes in between, to avoid overheating. Scrape down any mixture stuck to the sides of the pot.

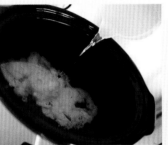

Step 4: Lumpy, gloopy cream soap mixture – this is quite normal!

Step 5
Place the smooth, very thick soap mixture back onto the heat and cook over a medium heat for 15 minutes. *Always* keep a lid on the mixture when it is being cooked and keep an eye on it in case it tries to separate. If it does separate, bring it back together with the stick blender.

Step 6
Reduce the heat and cook for a further one and a half to two hours. Stir every 30 minutes, taking care when inserting the spoon in case the mixture puffs up. If it does, stir with a long-handled spoon, allowing any trapped air to escape. Replace the lid and continue cooking. You may find it easier to chop into the spongy soap mixture with your spoon when it becomes too thick to stir.

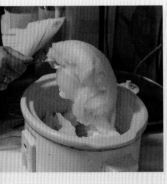

Step 6: Cream soap paste is very thick

Step 7
Once the mixture has a translucent glossy appearance rather like Vaseline, it is ready. Carry out a pH test using pH stripes, a pH meter or phenolphthalein. Refer to 'How to perform a phenolphthalein test' (page 144) for more details. If the cream soap is still a little on the alkali side, cook it for longer until you have a pH of about 7.

Step 8

Your cream soap is now very thick and will require diluting a little. Weigh the cream soap mixture to gauge how much water you need to add. There is no rule as to how much water to use since it depends on the consistency you require. Start by adding one-quarter of the cream soap's weight in water (for example, if your cream soap weighs 600 g, add 150 g hot water). If you wish to supercream your soap, add up to 5 per cent of the soap weight in melted stearic acid and/or glycerine. Warm these through first before adding to the cream soap. To give your cream soap a shelf life of 18 months or so, add your preferred preservative at this stage too. The shelf life of the soap is four months without a preservative and up to 18 months with a preservative.

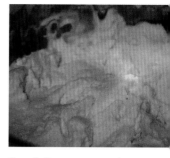

Step 8: Cream soap ready to be diluted

Place the cream soap, supercreaming ingredients and hot water in a large bowl or saucepan and use a handheld electric whisk to whisk the soap and water together. Keep whisking until you have a frothy, creamy consistency. If the mixture is too stiff, add a little more hot water to loosen it up and then whisk some more. Don't over-whisk it, since the soap will then become very light froth. The bubbles in the froth will dissipate after a while, leaving you with a thin soapy product.

Step 9

Put the whisked creamed soap into a lidded container and leave to rest for three or four weeks. This resting phase is known as 'rotting'. During the rotting stage the soap will become milder and more glossy, with a pearly sheen.

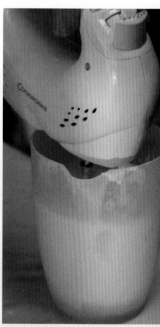

Step 8: Whisking cream soap will add volume and lightness

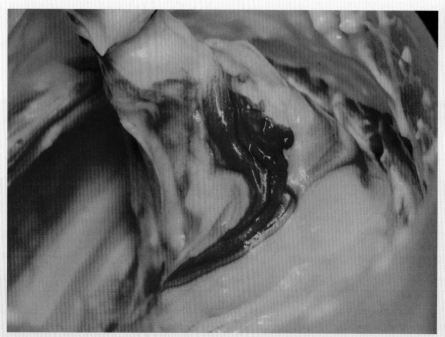

Step 10: The white cream soap can be coloured subtly or with bright and bold colours

Step 10

When the rotting phase is complete, remove some of the soap mixture to a separate bowl and add a little colour and up to 2 per cent essential or fragrance oil.

You can also add other functional ingredients such as rhassoul or clay to create a shaving soap, or sugar or salt to make an exfoliating soap.

RECIPES FOR CREAM SOAP

The recipes given on the following pages will yield approximately 2 litres creamy soap product, although you may find you have a lot more or less depending on how aerated the cream soap becomes when you whisk it.

Refer to the more detailed stages earlier in this section for a full description of the steps you need to make your cream soap. Make sure that you adhere to all the safety guidelines and wear protective clothing when making and handling your lye (pages 9–12).

I haven't included a preservative in my recipes, but if you wish to add one, please do so when adding your supercreaming ingredients and diluting your soap. Each preservative has different usage rates – some require 0.2 per cent and others up to 1.5 per cent, just follow the manufacturer's advice.

If you plan to sell your cream soap then a preservative is a good idea to give it an extended shelf life.

DESIGNING YOUR OWN CREAM SOAP RECIPES

Many of the soap calculators previously mentioned in this book will calculate hard bars and liquid soap but not cream soap. The best calculator to do this for you is the advanced soap calculator at www.summerbeemeadow.com. When designing your own cream soap recipes, you will need to know the formula for the amount of stearic acid and glycerine you should include.

The stearic acid is added at approximately twice the weight of oils. In the recipes given, I have used 140 g oils. If I multiply 140 by 2, this equals 280. Therefore I need to include approximately 280 g stearic acid, although a little more or a little less is fine too.

The glycerine is added at approximately one third of the weight of the oils and stearic acid added together. Using the calculation above, my oils weigh 140 g and the stearic acid weighs 280 g. If I add them together, they total 420 g. To find the weight of glycerine, I need to divide 420 g by 3, which equals 140 g. Therefore for each of my recipes I need approximately 140 g glycerine, but a little less or a little more will be fine.

Softly, softly, floating fun soap

This was a favourite in our household when the children were younger since they loved floating the soap on top of the bath water. Strawberry was voted the best!

LYE SOLUTION
14 g sodium hydroxide • 70 g potassium hydroxide • 370 g water

CREAM SOAP OILS, STEARIC ACID AND GLYCERINE
25 g sweet almond oil • 50 g olive oil • 40 g coconut oil
25 g shea butter • 275 g stearic acid • 140 g glycerine

DILUTION
Approximately 200 g warm water

SUPERCREAM INGREDIENTS
20 g stearic acid • 51 g glycerine

COLOURING
Red liquid colour

SCENT
20 g strawberry fragrance oil

METHOD
Refer to the cream making steps earlier in this section (pages 154–157) for further details.

In a saucepan, melt the oils and shea butter with the stearic acid.

Make up your lye by adding the sodium and potassium hydroxides to water and stir until the hydroxides have dissolved. Be sure to adhere to all the safety instructions (pages 9–12).

Remove the melted oils and stearic acid from the heat and add the glycerine.

Add the lye to the melted oils mixture and stir using a stick blender. Alternate between stick blender, spoon and resting until the cream soap has reached a thick, smooth trace.

Place the thick cream soap mixture back onto the heat and cook over a medium heat for 15 minutes.

Reduce the heat and cook for one and a half hours or until the mixture takes on a translucent, glossy appearance.

Test the pH (page 144) to make sure that the cream soap is cooked.

Add approximately 200 g warm water to your cream soap mixture. Melt the supercream stearic acid; add this and the supercream glycerine to the cream soap mixture. If you wish to add preservative, do so now.

Using a handheld electric whisk, mix the ingredients together until you have a creamy soap. Put the soap into a lidded container and leave to rest for three to four weeks.

Put the now-softened cream soap into a large bowl and add a few drops of red liquid colouring with the strawberry fragrance oil and mix. Place your cream soap in an individual lidded container.

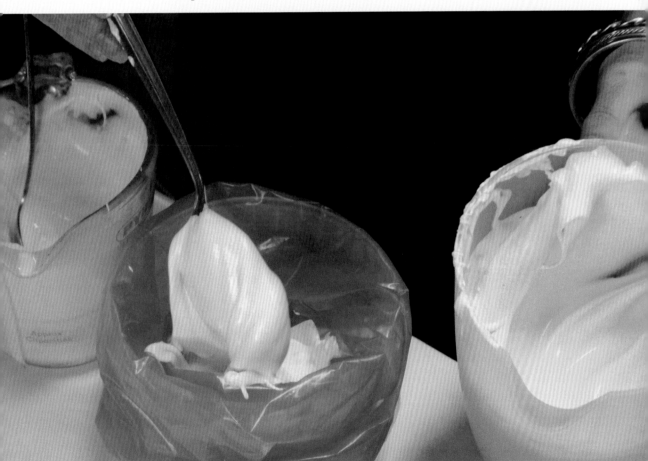

Potting up the Softly, softly floating fun soap

Purity shaving soap

Rich and luxurious, creamy soap makes the perfect shaving soap. I have added a little rhassoul, which will give a good slip when dragging the razor across the skin. I've also included aloe vera as part of the dilution to soothe and cool any overshaven patches.

LYE SOLUTION
59 g potassium hydroxide • 12 g sodium hydroxide • 310 g water

CREAM SOAP OILS, STEARIC ACID AND GLYCERINE
25 g coconut oil • 25 g castor oil • 25 g shea butter
20 g jojoba oil • 225 g stearic acid • 120 g glycerine

DILUTION
Approximately 100 g warm water • 100 g aloe vera

SUPERCREAM INGREDIENTS
18 g stearic acid • 45 g glycerine

SCENT
10 g lavender essential oil • 2 g vetiver essential oil

SOAP ADDITION
20 g rhassoul

METHOD
Follow the instructions for the Softly, softly floating fun soap recipe (page 158) and refer to the cream soap making steps (pages 154–157) for more detail. Add the aloe vera with the dilution (this can be added cold). Add the rhassoul at the same time as you add the essential oils.

Butter body cream soap

Cream soap is luxurious and creamy on its own, but I have added both shea and cocoa butters to this recipe to make it even more superb. This time half the dilution water has been substituted with rose water but you can use another floral water if you wish.

LYE SOLUTION
65 g potassium hydroxide • 13 g sodium hydroxide • 346 g water

CREAM SOAP OILS, STEARIC ACID AND GLYCERINE
20 g shea butter • 20 g cocoa butter • 40 g rice bran oil
40 g olive oil • 20 g coconut oil • 250 g stearic acid • 125 g glycerine

DILUTION
Approximately 100 g warm water • 100 g rose floral water

SUPERCREAM INGREDIENTS
19 g stearic acid • 48 g glycerine

SCENT
10 g rose fragrance oil • 10 g rose geranium essential oil

COLOUR
Pink liquid colouring

METHOD
Follow the instructions for the Softly, softly floating fun soap (page 158) recipe and refer to the cream soap making steps for more detail (pages 154–157). Add the rose water with the dilution (this can be added cold).

Silky body scrub

This is so delicious and what better way to spend your time in the shower than washing and exfoliating at the same time? I've added a little cyclomethicone to give the cream soap extra glide and a silky feel, but you can replace this with water if you don't have any. Both cyclomethicone and bamboo powder can be obtained from Plush Folly (see Resources at the back of this book), as well as other cosmetic ingredient suppliers.

This recipe also makes a fabulous exfoliating soap for dirty hands – the bamboo powder helps to rub away any stubborn dirt.

LYE SOLUTION
59 g potassium hydroxide • 12 g sodium hydroxide • 304 g water

CREAM SOAP OILS, STEARIC ACID AND GLYCERINE
50 g peach kernel oil • 40 g mango butter • 50 g avocado oil
225 g stearic acid • 125 g glycerine

DILUTION
Approximately 175 g warm water • 25 g cyclomethicone

SUPERCREAM INGREDIENTS
18 g stearic acid • 45 g glycerine

SCENT
5 g bergamot essential oil • 5 g mandarin essential oil
5 g juniper essential oil • 5 g patchouli essential oil

COLOUR
A few drops of liquid blue

ADDITION
40 g bamboo powder

METHOD
Follow the instructions for the Softly, softly floating fun soap recipe (page 158) and refer to the cream soap making steps (pages 154–157) for more detail. Add the cyclomethicone with the dilution (this can be added cold). At the same time as you add the essential oils, add the bamboo powder and mica. If you want a more robust, exfoliating product, double the amount of bamboo powder.

Silky body scrub cream soap

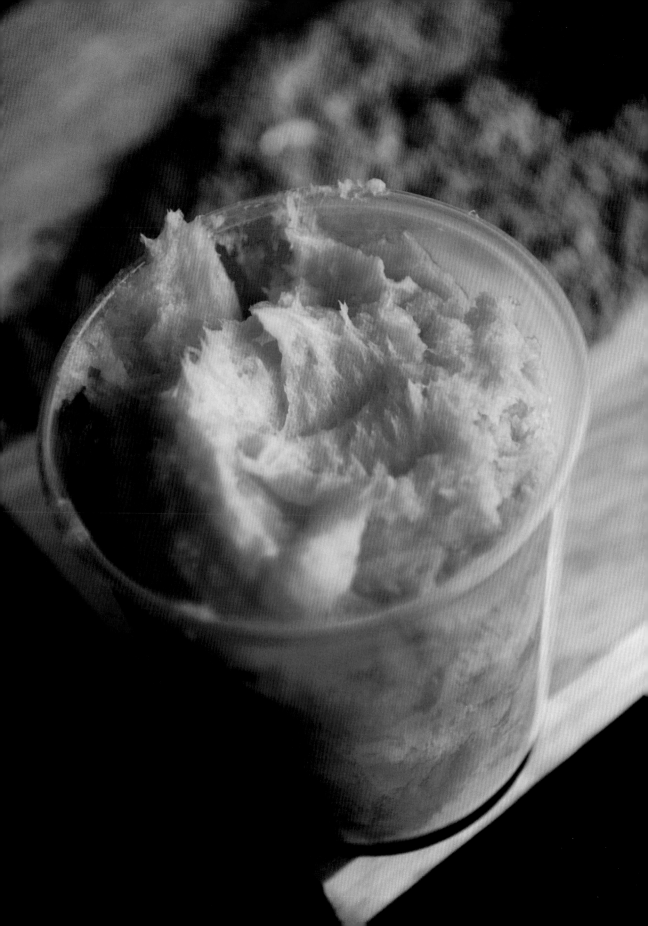

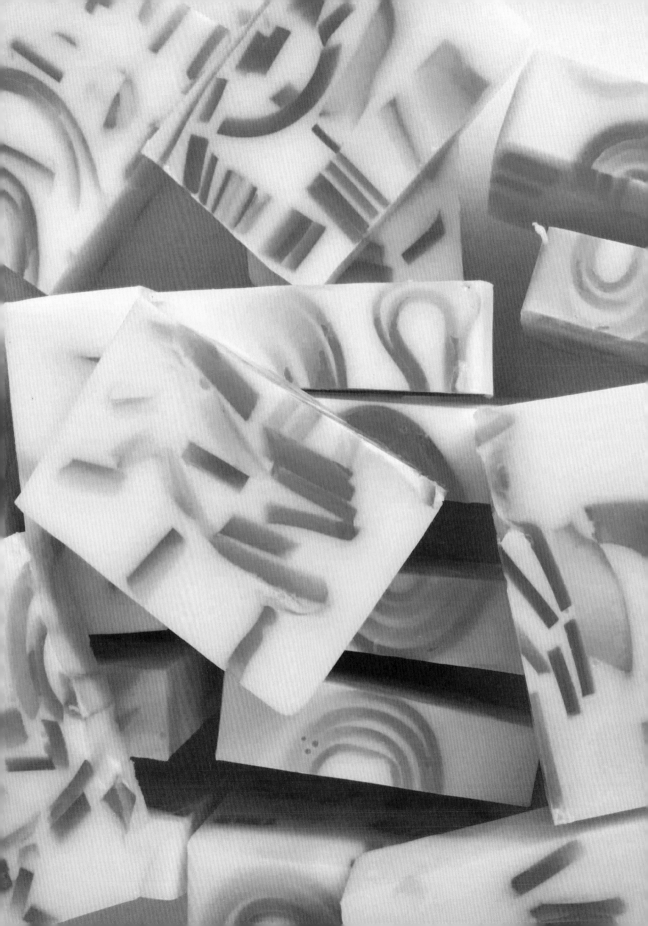

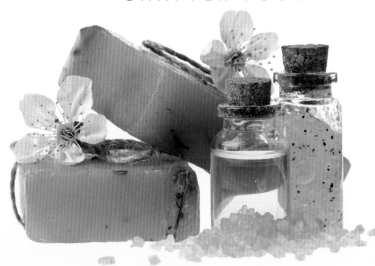

Crafting bars of soap using melt-and-pour soap base

For those who prefer not to start their soap making experience using sodium and potassium hydroxides, I have included a section on making melt-and-pour soaps. These are made from a base that you can buy ready-made. The soap base requires melting so that you can add colour and fragrance before pouring it into moulds to set – hence its name.

If you have an artistic streak, crafting with melt-and-pour soap can really get those creative juices flowing! Whilst many soap traditionalists prefer to use the 100 per cent natural lye soap making methods, melt-and-pour soap bases enable you to play around with colours, micas and glitters, bending, twisting, curling and embedding objects into or onto your soaps. The visual effects can be quite stunning. In the UK, there are two main manufacturers of soap bases. These are Leeds-based Stephensons, who make the Crystal range and Kays (based in Ramsbottom, Lancashire), who produce a range called Claranol.

If you wish to have a go at making your own melt-and-pour soap base, I have included instructions at the end of this section (page 194).

Melt-and-pour soap with
lemongrass embeds

SAFETY WHEN HANDLING MELT-AND-POUR SOAP BASE

Unlike traditional lye soaps, melt-and-pour soap bases do not contain any ingredients that may be considered hazardous. However, since the soap base will need to be heated in order for it to melt, you will be handling it at a temperature of approximately 70°C (158°F) and all due care should be taken not to burn yourself.

WHAT IS MELT-AND-POUR SOAP BASE?

Soap has traditionally been made using a combination of lye, water and a blend of fats, oils and butters. However, the use of lye – a potentially hazardous ingredient – deters many would-be soap makers. With melt-and-pour soap bases, the processing of the lye and oils has already been carried out for you so that the soap base is safe to handle. Extra ingredients have been added to the bases to ensure they have a long shelf life, feel silky and moisturising on the skin, remain hard even when wet, create a good foam, clean the skin and so on.

Melt-and-pour soap base is a manufactured base made up of a number of different ingredients designed to produce a hard bar that lathers up quickly and easily whilst feeling gentle and kind on the skin – and it washes too! It contains glycerine, which is a humectant. A humectant will draw moisture from the air and lock it onto the skin's surface, helping it to remain hydrated for longer. Melt-and-pour soap is often known as 'glycerine soap' due to its high glycerine content.

SHELF LIFE OF MELT-AND-POUR SOAPS

Finished melt-and-pour soaps will have a shelf life of at least two years although the colour and fragrance may fade a little as the soap ages.

Different types of melt-and-pour soap base

There are several different types of soap base available. The basic and most frequently used soap bases include opaque and clear soap bases (often referred to as 'white' and 'transparent' bases). Clear soap bases can be coloured and fragranced and will mostly retain their clarity. Some essential or fragrance oils may make the soap base slightly cloudy, as may the addition of any extra oils.

The opaque soap base is the same as the clear soap base, but with the addition of titanium dioxide, a natural white colouring used extensively in cosmetics. This soap base can also be coloured, but the white base colour must be taken into consideration. For example, adding a red colouring will initially make the soap go pink.

White melt-and-pour soap base

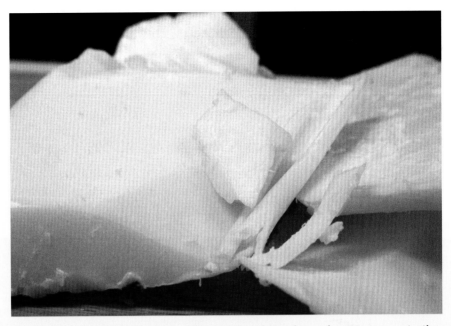

The ingredients for both the Stephensons' and Kays' soap bases are very similar. The Claranol clear soap base ingredients (Kays) are listed as follows:

Aqua • Propylene glycol • Sodium stearate • Sodium laureth sulphate • Glycerine Sucrose • Sodium Cocoate • Sodium xylene sulphonate • Sodium lauryl sulphate Stearic acid • Tetrasodium EDTA • Tetrasodium etidronate

The Stephensons' clear soap base ingredients are listed as follows:

Aqua • Glycerin • Sodium Stearate • Propylene Glycol • Sorbitol Sodium Laurate • Sodium Laureth Sulfate • Sodium Lauryl Sulfate Sodium Chloride • Stearic Acid • Lauric Acid • Pentasodium Pentetate Tetrasodium Etidronate

In addition to these basic bases, there are soap bases that are made with organic oils or that contain mostly natural ingredients, a base that is SLS (sodium lauryl sulphate) free, a base that doesn't 'sweat', a base offering better clarity, a base that will allow the suspension of glitter and other particles, a base that makes a particularly good shaving soap, a base suitable for use as a solid shampoo, and bases with the addition of goats' milk, olive oil, honey, shea butter, aloe vera or other beneficial cosmetic ingredients.

Rather than use a base with added ingredients, it is possible to add your own ingredients, such as olive oil, jojoba oil, aloe vera, and so on to the melted soap base. However, do not add more than 5 per cent of the soap base weight as the soap will become too wet, sticky or soft. Please note: soaps with added oils, butters and other ingredients are likely to be a little cloudy.

The recipes in this section can be made using whichever soap base you prefer, but you will need to choose appropriate clear or opaque bases if you wish to do some of the special effects.

Regardless of which soap base you choose, the method of melting, colouring, fragrancing and crafting your soap will be the same.

Equipment needed for making melt-and-pour soaps

No specialist equipment is necessary and quite possibly, you already have everything you need, although it is worth collecting a dedicated soap-making toolkit rather than using your kitchen equipment. The equipment you will need includes:

- Heatproof jug(s) or saucepans (plastic ones are fine for use in the microwave)
- Big saucepans (if planning to melt your soap base on the hob)
- Stainless steel spoons for stirring
- A set of digital scales to weigh the soap base
- Moulds of various sizes

MOULDS SUITABLE FOR MELT-AND-POUR SOAPS

Whilst there are some fabulous and funky shaped moulds available, you can save yourself some money by using all sorts of household items as soap moulds. Be sure to reserve them for soap making once used, though. I remember walking around our local supermarket eyeing up all sorts of packets of food,

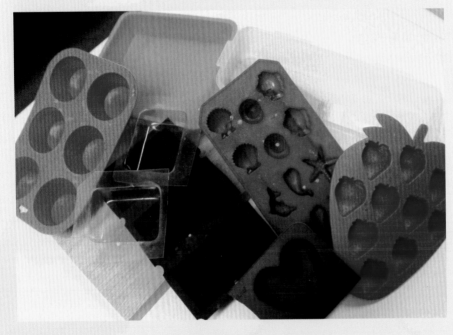

All sorts of specialist or household items can be used for moulding melt-and-pour soaps

trying to work out whether the empty containers could be used as a soap mould. The staff in there have since got used to me asking if I can take the empty trays that hold the double cream cartons in place, as the individual cavities make wonderful moulds.

Ice-cube trays

I have a huge selection of novelty ice-cube trays that enable me to make tiny soaps in all sorts of shapes – shells, starfish, fish, ducks, shoes, handbags, stars, hearts, pieces of jigsaw, smiley faces and more. Rubber, silicone or rigid plastic ones will do, but the flexible silicone trays are the easiest to use.

Chocolate moulds

Chocolate moulds make great guest soaps and small soaps to embed in larger bars. These can be found online and in specialist cookery shops.

Yoghourt pots

Make sure your pot is clean and dry before using it. Also, be careful not to pour the soap in while it is too hot in case it melts the pot.

Blister packs

A blister pack is the pre-formed transparent plastic packaging often attached to a piece of cardboard used to package small consumable items such as computer accessories and small toys. If you are lucky enough, you can remove the item without breaking the blister pack. And if you are even luckier, it will be the perfect shape for soap!

Silicone bread and cake moulds

Silicone moulds intended for bread or cakes make ideal large soap moulds. You can cut your set soap into slices as you would a cake or a loaf of bread. Whilst metal cake or bread tins may be used, they will need to be lined with cling film or similar to make it easier to remove the soap from the mould.

Food containers

Empty, washed-out and dried juice cartons, crisp tubes, ice-cream tubs and similar are all perfect for use as a soap mould. If the container is made of plastic you will be able to reuse it, but if it is cardboard (like the crisp tube) then it will be a single-use mould, as it is likely that you will need to cut and peel the mould away from the soap. My children never seem to mind when I ask them to eat crisps so that I can have several moulds available!

Preparing your melt-and-pour soap base for use

The soap base will need to be cut into small chunks to make it quick to melt, so reducing the risk of burning. Cut the soap up and place it in a pan (if melting on the hob) or put it in a heatproof jug and melt in a microwave using 30-second bursts of high heat.

Remove from the heat and stir well to ensure all the chunks of soap base are melted. It is possible to overheat and burn your soap base so never leave it unattended or heat it for a prolonged time at high temperatures. Not only is this dangerous, you will have to start all over again as the base will be brown and smell of burnt soap.

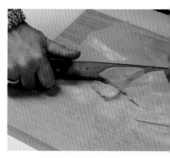

Cutting the transparent melt-and-pour soap base ready for melting

The soap base can be remelted – even when it has been coloured and fragranced. This means that there is very little wastage.

Fragrancing your melt-and-pour soap base

You can use both essential and fragrance oils in your melt-and-pour soap base. Both are reliable and will not cause any adverse reaction in your soap, although some oils may cause a little discolouration.

Essential and fragrance oils are typically added at 2 per cent, although since the soap holds its aroma very well, you may find that 1 per cent is plenty. See the section on calculating percentages (page 26) to work out how much fragrance you should add.

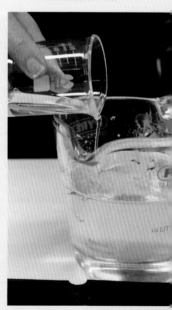

Melting the clear melt-and-pour soap base

If you add the oils when the soap is still very hot you will lose some of the aroma's potency. Wait until the soap is cooling a little before you add the oil, but not so cool that it is starting to solidify.

Drip or pour the essential or fragrance oil into the melted soap base and stir well. Do not stir too wildly or you will create bubbles that will remain when you pour your melted soap into the moulds. *Always* add the fragrance or essential oils before adding the colour. Each essential or fragrance oil has its own slight colour tinge, which will have an effect on the colour you choose for your soap. Adding the colour after the fragrance or essential oils takes into account the oil colour tinge.

Colouring the melt-and-pour soap base

There are many different formats of coloured ingredients that you can use to add a tint to your finished soap. Below is a brief guide to these options.

LIQUID COLOURS

Similar to food colouring, liquid cosmetic colours are very intense. A little goes a long way, so do not be tempted to add too much. Start with a drop or two and stir well to incorporate the colour into the soap. Add a little more, drop by drop, until you have obtained the required shade.

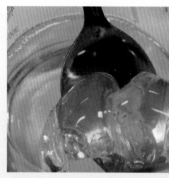

Adding fragrance oil to your clear melt-and-pour soap base

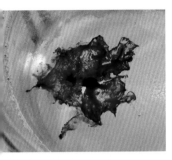

Adding liquid colour to the melted melt-and-pour soap base

WATER-SOLUBLE POWDERED COLOURS

When using powdered colours you may find it easier to mix the powder in a little warm water or oil first. This helps to break down and disperse the colour and prevents speckles of undispersed colour appearing in your finished soap. If your powdered colour is oil-soluble, blend it with a little oil before adding it to the soap base to help prevent speckles of colour occurring. With water-soluble powdered colours mix with a little water before adding to the soap base.

To determine whether your powder is water or oil-soluble, place about 50 ml water into a glass and sprinkle a little powdered colour on top. Stir well. If the powder dissolves into the water, then it is water-soluble; if the powder particles suspend or sink to the bottom then it is not water-soluble and may be oil-soluble. Repeat the exercise using oil instead of water to double-check that the coloured particles disperse evenly in oil.

USING MICA

Mica will add a shimmering effect to your soap and can look beautiful. It works far better in transparent soap than the opaque soap base, although it will make the soap cloudy. If used in opaque soap base, the soap will be coloured but won't show the beautiful metallic shimmering effect as much.

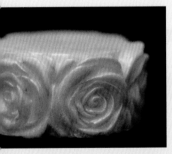

Gold mica has added a subtle, but beautiful shimmer to this white soap

COLOUR DEPTH

The more colour you add, the darker your soaps will become, but do be careful not to add so much that your flannels and towels stain from any un-rinsed soapy residue.

Adding colour to the white soap base will give you a pastel shade whilst adding colour to the clear soap base gives a stronger shade. You can mix the clear and white soap bases together to get different depths of colour shades. For example, if you combine 400 g clear soap base with 50 g white soap base, the uncoloured soap will look as though you have used only white soap base. However, when you add a drop or two of colour, the finished result will be much stronger in the combined soap bases than in the white soap base.

POURING YOUR MELT-AND-POUR SOAP

When the soap base has melted and you have added your fragrance and colour, it is ready to be poured into moulds. Pour gently to avoid having bubbles trapped inside or resting on your finished bars of soap.

If you do find you have bubbles on the surface, spraying with a gentle mist of surgical spirits or rubbing alcohol onto the soap immediately after you have poured it will help to remove the bubbles.

Leave the soap somewhere cool to set. Setting takes approximately two hours depending on whether you have made individual bars or are pouring a block of soap to cut later. Setting times can be speeded up (depending on the heat of soap and size of mould) by placing your soap in the fridge or freezer.

REMOVING YOUR MELT-AND-POUR SOAP FROM YOUR MOULDS

To take your soap out of a mould, turn the mould upside down and push the base as if pushing out a stubborn ice cube. If your mould is made of silicone, you can literally just peel the silicone away from the soap to release it.

If soap refuses to be dislodged from the mould, press down hard on the back of the mould with the heel of your hand. If it still refuses to budge, put the soap and mould in the freezer for 15 minutes or so – this causes the soap to shrink a tiny amount and it should pop out more easily.

As soon as they are out of the moulds, your soaps are ready for use. You do not need to use them straightaway as they will still be okay to use for at least 18 months after production.

Since the soap base has a high glycerine content it will draw moisture from the air. If left exposed to the air, it may start to form a layer of beads of moisture. This is known as the soap 'sweating'. The moisture does not have an adverse effect on the quality, benefits or use of the soap, but will make it wet and slippery. Wet droplets can be wiped off with a clean tissue. Once wrapped or stored in an airtight container, changes in the air temperature will not make the soap sweat. One of the soap bases mentioned earlier when I talk about the different types of melt-and-pour soap (pages 166–7) is a 'low-sweat' soap base, which eliminates the problem of having to wrap soaps to prevent sweating.

ADDING BOTANICALS TO YOUR SOAP BASE

Botanicals, such as dried herbs and petals, can be added to your soap to make it attractive and interesting. Note that over time, most herbs and petals will gradually turn brown, which can potentially make your soap less attractive than you planned! Soaps containing botanicals should not be used on the face as the botanicals may be slightly abrasive.

To add herbs and petals, first melt, colour and fragrance your soap base as usual. You will need to add the botanicals when the soap base is liquid, but not too hot. Carefully sprinkle in your chosen plant material and stir gently to disperse the petals or herbs evenly throughout the soap.

Do not be tempted to add too much – you are trying to create a pretty bar of soap rather than a bar of soap that will mean you have to clean the bath or shower after using it! We usually add between half and one teaspoon of botanical per 100 g soap base, but less is good too.

Transparent pink soap with rose petals

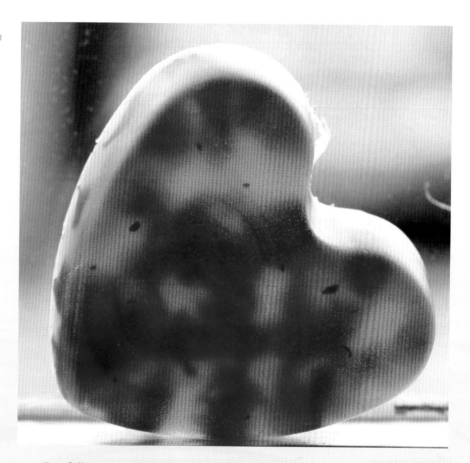

Carefully pour your soap mixture into the moulds. If the soap base is too hot when you pour it, the botanicals will not be suspended in the melted soap mixture and will sink to the bottom of your mould. Unless you particularly wanted them evenly distributed throughout the soap, this might no matter and will quite possibly look more attractive (go on, convince yourself!). However, to prevent the botanicals from sinking, leave the soap mixture to cool a little (but not to the point where it is trying to set) before pouring it into the moulds.

The 'suspending' soap base will help to suspend the botanicals evenly throughout the soap rather than allow them to sink.

Adding clays and powders to your soap base

Coloured clays and powders can be added to your soap not only to give colour, but to give additional benefit to your skin too. Although soap is a rinse-off product and not in direct contact with the skin for long, certain benefits can be derived from including skin-enhancing minerals in your soaps.

I recommend mixing the clays or powders with a little warm water initially. This will help to ensure that they blend into the soap base without creating unwanted lumps or speckles. Simply mix a teaspoon or so of the powder with a couple of teaspoons of warm water and stir to create a slurry. Add the slurry to your melted soap base and stir well. Note: using warm water rather than cold will help to keep the soap mixture liquid whilst you stir.

Ingredient	Benefit (apart from adding colour)
Clays such as kaolin clay, bentonite clay and Fuller's Earth	Adds slip and glide to your soaps – especially useful if you are creating a shaving soap
Muds such as Dead Sea mud	Rich in minerals and deep cleansing
Mineral ashes such as rhassoul or pumice	Adds slip (rhassoul) and can be gently exfoliating (pumice), as well as introducing nutrients to the skin
Powdered seaweeds such as kelp or bladderwrack	Kelp and other seaweed is rich in skin strengthening minerals
Dairy powders such as goats' milk, buttermilk or yoghourt powder	Skin softening and helps give the soap a creamy feel

RECIPES FOR MELT-AND-POUR SOAP BASE

If you are crafty and enjoy being creative, you'll have so much fun designing and creating your own soaps. The recipes on the following pages include a range of ideas to get you started.

Orange marmalade soap

So called because someone once asked me if I had made this soap using marmalade – it doesn't contain marmalade but looks as if it might!

INGREDIENTS
300 g clear melt-and-pour soap base
6 g sweet orange essential oil
1–2 drops orange liquid colour
A few calendula (marigold) petals

METHOD
Melt the clear soap base, leave to cool a little before adding the sweet orange essential oil and orange colouring. Stir well and scatter a few calendula petals into the melted soap base. Stir gently to disperse the petals evenly throughout the soap.

Carefully pour into three 100 g soap moulds, making sure that the calendula petals remain suspended in the soap. Leave to set.

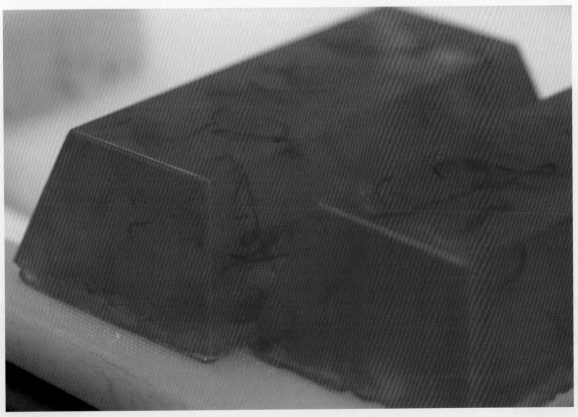

Orange marmalade soap

Gardener's scrubby soap

One of our most popular soaps, this has been sold at the Chelsea Flower Show and Hampton Court Flower Show with masses of repeat orders received. Due to the exfoliating properties of the pumice and seeds, this soap will help to remove any stubborn dirt after a hard session gardening. It also contains 5 per cent jojoba oil to soften and moisturise hands.

Ingredients
300 g opaque melt-and-pour soap base
6 g hemp fragrance oil • 1 drop green liquid colour
10 g jojoba oil • 5 g pumice • A few strawberry seeds

Method
Melt the soap base, leave to cool a little before adding the hemp fragrance oil and green colouring. Stir well. Pour the jojoba oil into a separate pot and stir in the pumice powder, stirring well to create a slurry. Add this slurry to the melted soap base and scatter a few strawberry seeds in as well.

Stir gently to disperse the seeds and pumice evenly throughout the soap. Carefully pour the mixture into three 100 g soap moulds, making sure that the seeds remain suspended in the soap. Leave to set.

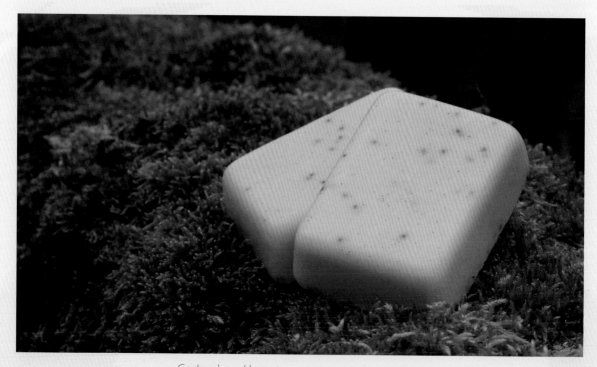

Gardener's scrubby soap

Midas butter bar

The gold mica adds a shimmer of gold, whilst the buttermilk gives skin softening properties. Teamed with the delicious aroma of vanilla bourbon, I defy you not to want to make and use this soap over and over again!

The vanillin content of the vanilla bourbon fragrance oil will slowly add a beige tint to your soap and it will turn a little darker over time. Gold mica will continue to give a subtle shimmer regardless of the stage of beige.

INGREDIENTS
300 g clear melt-and-pour soap base
6 g vanilla bourbon fragrance oil
1 g soft gold mica
5 g buttermilk powder

METHOD
Melt the clear soap base, add the vanilla bourbon fragrance oil and stir well. In a separate pot, add the gold mica and the buttermilk powder to one teaspoon hot water; stir to create a slurry.

Add the golden buttermilk slurry to the melted vanilla soap base and stir well. Pour into the moulds and leave to set.

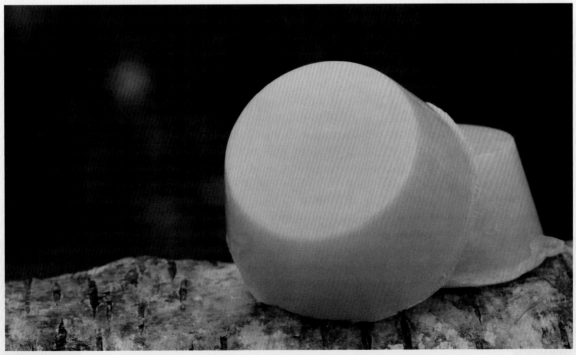

Midas butter bars

Special effects with melt-and-pour soap

One of the enormous benefits of using melt-and-pour soap is the absolutely stunning effects you can create. You can twist, layer, bend and shape soap, coat it in mica and glitter and embed it in transparent soap, embed objects, even print onto rice paper and embed messages in your soap. Melt-and-pour soap is the perfect medium for all kinds of surprises!

LAYERING DIFFERENT COLOURED MELT-AND-POUR SOAP

Layering different colours of melt-and-pour soap is very simple and looks extremely attractive. All you need is a mould, two different coloured soap bases and some isopropyl alcohol.

Pour your first coloured, fragranced layer into the mould and give it a squirt with isopropyl alcohol to remove any surface bubbles. Leave it to set. If you are in a hurry, you can pour the second layer without the first layer setting, but you will get better results if you leave it to set hard. Carefully prod the first layer with a clean finger to make sure that it isn't still soft and melted. If it yields slightly to the touch but feels solid, then it is ready for the second layer. Alternatively leave for an hour or so until it has definitely set hard. Before pouring the second soap base, give the first layer another squirt with isopropyl alcohol to encourage adhesion between the two layers. Make sure that the second base is not hot enough to melt the first layer by checking with a clean finger as above, then carefully pour onto the first layer. Leave to set.

Layering soap in this way needn't be limited to two layers – I have seen beautiful 'rainbow' coloured soap with seven different colour layers. Just make sure that you squirt with isopropyl alcohol before pouring in a new layer and that the pouring soap isn't hot enough to melt the previous one.

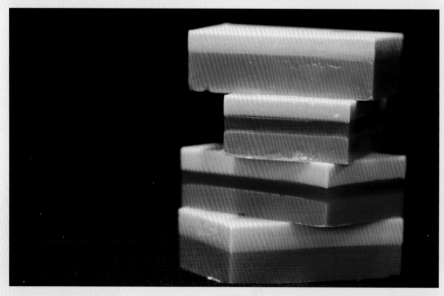

Pink and burgundy layer soap

Liquorice layer soap

Black soap can be very messy and you must be careful not to add too much black in case any soapy residue discolours your towels. It is the perfect colour for our glorious aniseed essential oil and what better way to use it, but in a stripy soap! The strawberry fragrance oil in the pink part of the soap reminds me of the smell of sweet, strawberry liquorice laces from my childhood.

INGREDIENTS
50 g clear melt-and-pour soap base
250 g opaque melt-and-pour soap base
$^1/_4$–$^1/_2$ teaspoon black mica • 2 g aniseed essential oil
4 g strawberry fragrance oil • 3 or 4 drops red liquid colour

METHOD
Melt both the soap bases in separate containers.

To a small heatproof jug or bowl, add a tiny amount of hot water to the black mica and swill it around to create a mostly black, watery solution. Pour the clear soap base onto this black mixture and then add about 5 g opaque soap base to the clear soap base – this prevents the black part of your soap from being transparent. Don't add any more than 10 g or you will create a grey colour rather than black. If it looks a little grey, add more black mica to a little hot water and blend into the soap mixture. Add the aniseed essential oil and stir well.

Add the strawberry fragrance oil to the opaque melt-and-pour base and stir well. Remove about 50 g opaque strawberry soap base and place in a little heatproof jug or bowl. Set this to one side.

Add the red liquid colour to the remaining opaque strawberry soap base to turn it pink and stir well. Now that you have your soap bases coloured and fragranced, you are ready for the first pour. The soap bases will set in the heatproof jugs before you are ready to pour all the layers. To re-melt simply pop the jug into a microwave on low or medium for a minute or two before you need to pour it. Note: although microwaving on high will also work, there is a risk of burning if it is left in too long.

Choose which colour you would like to start with (remember, if your soap mould is such that you pour your soap upside down, this will become the top layer of soap). Pour a thin layer of this soap into the mould and spritz with isopropyl alcohol. Leave it to set.

When the first layer is hard enough to hold the weight of your second layer, spritz again and then carefully pour in the second layer. Spritz the second layer with isopropyl alcohol.

Continue building your layered soap, spritzing each layer once you have poured it and again before you add another layer on top of it. Leave the layered soaps to set.

Liquorice layer soap

EMBEDDING ITEMS IN SOAP

Small objects such as novelty rubbers, items of jewellery and beads can all be placed in a soap mould and carefully covered in clear soap base, embedding them safely until you wash enough times to release them from their soapy prison. I always fancied making the world's most expensive bar of soap by embedding a very expensive diamond ring – I just didn't have the money for the diamond in the first place!

Do remember that these soaps are not suitable for small children as the object may be a choking hazard.

Embedding objects is easy. Using the instructions already described in this section, make up a sufficient quantity of lightly coloured and fragranced clear soap base. Don't add too much colour – you want to be able to see the embedded object through the soap.

Pour a thin layer of this soap base into your mould. Carefully place your novelty object onto the base, making sure that you have it the right way up. Remember that some moulds result in the soap being made upside down so that the bottom of the mould becomes the top of the soap – if this is the type

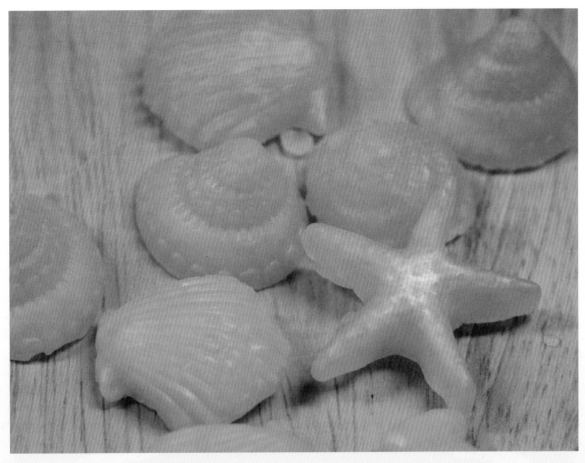

Soapy sea shells and starfish embeds

of mould you are using, your embedded object needs to be placed face down in the mould. Spray a quick squirt of isopropyl alcohol (or rubbing alcohol) onto the thin soap layer to help the next layer that you are about to pour adhere well.

When the first, thin layer has formed a skin and has started to set, very carefully pour more of the clear soap base over the soap layer and embedded object so that the mould is filled to the top. Make sure that the second soap base is not hot enough to melt the first layer of soap – this is all a question of look and feel, and experience.

The embedded object may move or float to the top of the soap. To prevent this happening, hold it in place with a cocktail stick or similar. Leave the cocktail stick in the soap until you are sure that the setting process has started. After a few minutes, carefully remove the cocktail stick by giving it a little twist whilst gently pulling it out of the soap.

EMBEDDING SOAP IN SOAP

Rather than embed novelty objects, you can also make your own soapy embeds to place in soap. To make tiny soap shapes, you will need a novelty ice-cube tray, chocolate moulds or similar.

Making soap embeds

Make up a batch of opaque melt-and-pour soap base (page 170). Add your chosen colour and fragrance then pour into ice-cube trays or chocolate moulds. When the soaps are set, remove the shapes from the moulds and place in the fridge or freezer to chill until cold (about 15 minutes). If I don't need the shapes straightaway, I will leave them chilling for days.

Meanwhile, melt and lightly colour and fragrance your transparent soap base (page 170). Pour a thin layer of slightly cooled, but still molten soap into the moulds. Spritz with isopropyl alcohol to ensure the soapy embed will stick to the other layers. Leave the soap to set (about 15 minutes). Remove your embed shapes from the mould in the fridge or freezer and carefully lay one on each of the thin layers of soap, being careful to place them the right way up. Spritz the embed shapes with isopropyl alcohol and very carefully pour the remaining soap over the top, being careful not to dislodge the embed as you pour. You may wish to hold them in place with a cocktail stick (page 181). Once the soap has set, carefully remove the cocktail stick before removing the soap from the moulds.

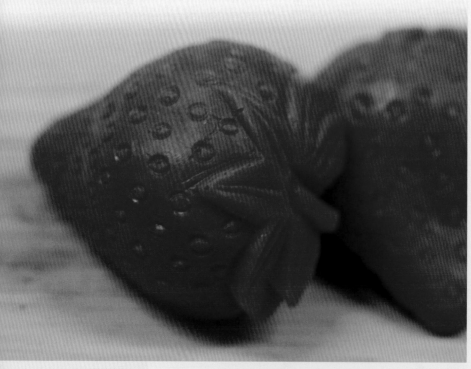

Strawberry soap embeds

Strawberry soap

For this recipe you will also need a strawberry shaped mould. I have used an ice-cube tray with strawberry shaped cavities.

INGREDIENTS

60 g opaque melt-and-pour soap base • 5 g strawberry fragrance oil
4 or 5 drops red liquid colouring • 200 g clear melt-and-pour soap base

METHOD

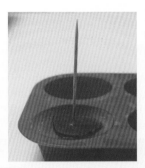

Use a cocktail stick to prevent the embed from floating in the soap

Melt the opaque soap base then leave to cool a little before adding 1 g strawberry fragrance oil and the red liquid colouring. Stir well. Pour the red, strawberry-scented soap into the strawberry shaped moulds and leave to set (about 15 minutes). When the strawberry shapes have set, remove from the mould and pop them into the fridge.

Melt the clear soap base and add the remaining 4 g strawberry fragrance oil, stirring well. Pour a thin layer into your soap moulds and leave to set.

Remove the strawberry shapes from the fridge and give each one a squirt with isopropyl alcohol. Place a strawberry shape on the thin, clear layer of set soap base (you may need to insert a cocktail stick into the base of the strawberry shape to hold it upright and to prevent it from falling onto its side).Carefully pour the clear, strawberry-scented soap base over the strawberry shape. Fill to the top of the mould, immersing the strawberry shape in transparent soap. Carefully twist and remove the cocktail stick when the soap has started to set. Leave the soaps to set completely (about 15 minutes) before removing them from the mould.

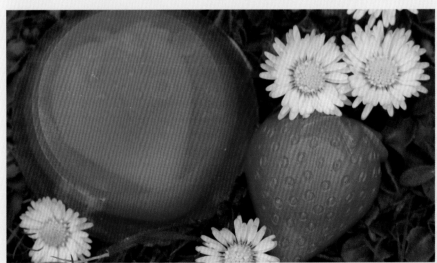

Strawberry soap

MAKING SOAP TWISTS AND SPIRALS

There is something very therapeutic about bending and shaping soap. I love twisting soap around my chopsticks or fingers to produce coils, twirls and swirls. The final soaps can be beautiful, although somewhat unpredictable!

In order to create bends and twists you need to start off with a sheet of recently poured soap that is still on the soft side. A plastic tray, lunch box or clean 1-litre ice-cream carton make the perfect mould for your sheet of soap.

To make a sheet of soap, melt, fragrance and colour your soap base as usual (page 170) and then pour a 1 cm layer of soap base into your chosen mould. Leave until set, but only just set. Carefully lift one corner of the soap from the

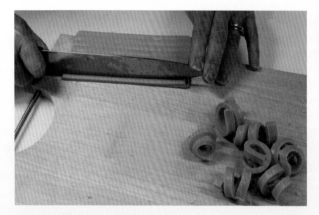

Cutting strips to make soap curls

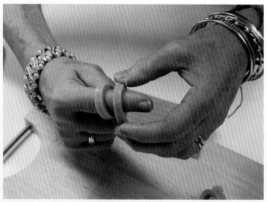

Wrap the soap strips around your finger to create a soap curl

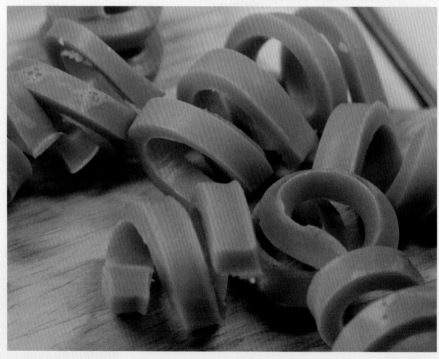

Blue soap swirls ready to be embedded in soap

mould and then peel away the entire sheet of soap. Place the soap sheet on a chopping board and cut a thin slither from one edge.

Take the thin slither of soap and wrap it around a chopstick, a pencil, pen or even your finger so that it bends into a coil shape. Carefully remove the coil and place to one side. Repeat with the remaining soap sheet until you have a pile of coiled soap.

As well as coils, you can create bends by cutting a strip of soap and bending it into a wriggly 'S' shape – just let your creative imagination run riot!

Peel thin curls of soap by slowly pulling a vegetable peeler down the longer edge of your soap sheet. As you peel you will produce a thin ribbon of curled soap, which can be embedded in soap.

EMBEDDING YOUR CURLS, TWISTS AND SPIRALS

Before placing your curls, twists and spirals into your soap mould, make sure you have sprayed a fine mist of isopropyl alcohol onto each shape to secure them.

Place the shape in your mould – either directly onto the base of the mould or onto a thin layer of previously poured soap. Carefully pour the outer soap layer over the twists, making sure that the outer soap layer is warm enough to pour but not so hot as to melt the twists. Note: the only way to check this is to pour and then watch and see if it melts.

Use a potato peeler to shave thin ribbons of curled soap

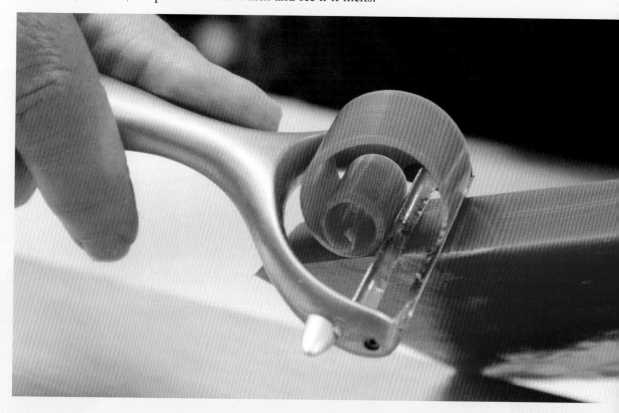

Rosy ribbons soap

One of the most girlie pink soaps ever! The pink curls of soap look like beautiful ribbons embedded in clear rose-fragranced soap. The clear outer soap gives a three-dimensional effect, making this soap even more gorgeous.

Ingredients
100 g opaque melt-and-pour soap base • 6 g tea rose fragrance oil
5 or 6 drops pink liquid colour • 280 g clear melt-and-pour soap base

Method
First, make your block of pink soap by melting the opaque melt-and-pour soap base and adding 2 g tea rose fragrance oil and 4 or 5 drops of pink colouring. Stir well and pour a thin 1–2 cm layer of soap into a mould.

When the soap block has set, remove from the mould. Using a clean potato peeler, carefully peel a thin layer of soap down the longest edge of the soap block. Peel slowly to enable the thin soap peel to naturally curl round itself.

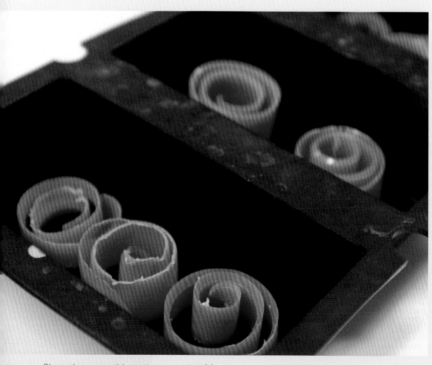

Place the soap ribbons into your mould

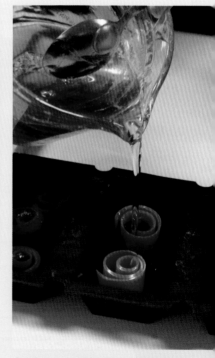

Carefully pour the melted soap over the soap ribbons

Repeat this process, peeling the soap into several thin, fragile curls. Carefully place the curls onto the base of your soap mould and place the mould into the fridge.

To make the body of the soap, melt the clear soap base and add the remaining tea rose fragrance oil. Add one drop of pink colour to the clear soap base and stir well. When the soap has cooled a little, but is still pourable, remove the mould with the curls in it from the fridge and give the curls a spritz of isopropyl alcohol.

Carefully pour the clear soap base over the curls, trying not to dislodge them as you pour. You can use a cocktail stick to help keep them in place but really, the whole effect is random. Leave to set then turn the soap out of the moulds.

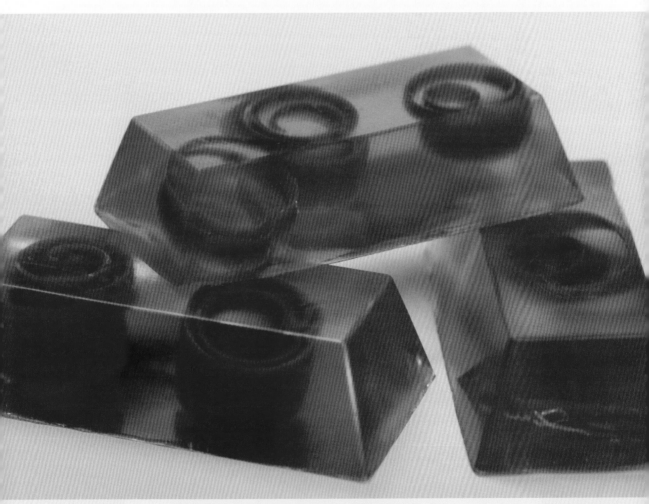

Rosy ribbons soap

Mango and strawberry swirl soap

Beautiful bars of mango and strawberry soap so delicious you'll wish they were edible. But it's not, so please don't even try licking the soap! This soap needs to be made into a loaf and cut in slices to get the full effect of the swirl. I have suggested 500 g opaque melt-and-pour soap base, but if your mould capacity is bigger or smaller than 500 g, adjust the amount of opaque soap base to suit. My recipe fragrances at 2 per cent, hence the 10 g mango fragrance oil, which is the right amount to fragrance 500 g soap base. Don't forget to adjust this amount too, if necessary.

INGREDIENTS
100 g clear melt-and-pour soap base • 2 g strawberry fragrance oil
4 drops red liquid colour • 500 g opaque melt-and-pour soap base
10 g mango fragrance oil

METHOD
Melt the clear soap and add 2 g strawberry fragrance oil and 3 drops red liquid colouring. Stir well and pour a 1 cm layer of the melted soap into a tray mould.

When the soap has just set, remove from the mould and bend the entire sheet of strawberry soap into a swirl. Spritz the strawberry swirl with isopropyl alcohol and place in your loaf mould, trimming any excess swirl so that it fits snugly into the mould. Place the soap mould and swirl in the fridge to chill (about 15 minutes). Melt the opaque soap base and add any excess strawberry red curl trimmings. Once melted, add the mango fragrance oil and stir well.

Remove the strawberry soap from the fridge and when the opaque mango soap base is cool enough to pour without melting the strawberry swirl, pour the mango soap over the swirl until it is immersed in the soap. Leave to set before chopping into slices. Note: the setting time depends on the size of mould and your pouring temperature. As a general guide, allow two hours in summer, less in winter.

*Mango and strawberry
swirl soap*

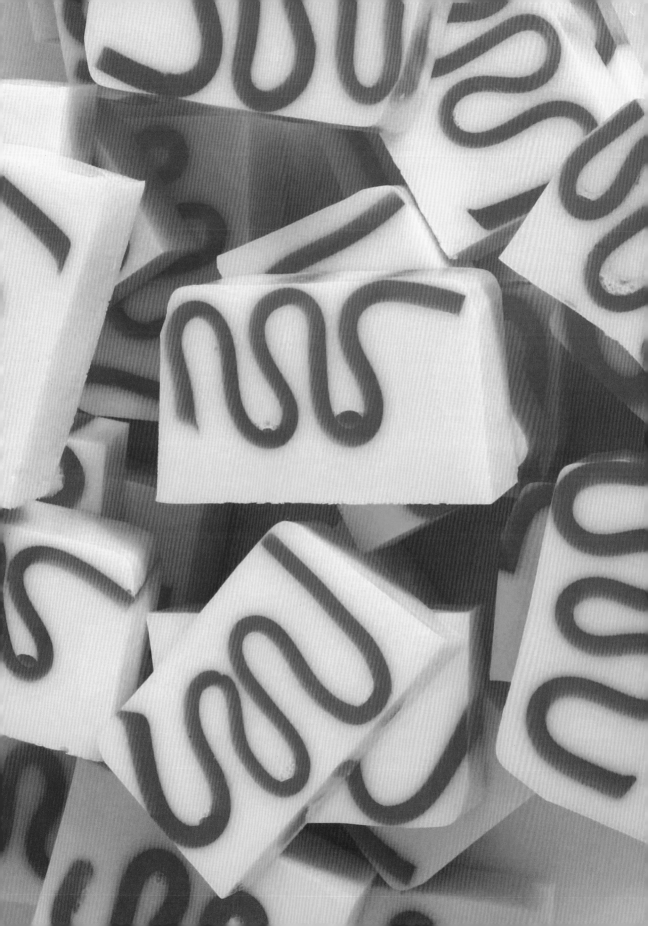

Blue, blue soap

Round soap seems to be a very popular shape and whilst I love making this particular soap, I always find wrapping a round shaped soap rather tricky. This is one of those soaps that looks almost too good to use!

INGREDIENTS
600 g clear melt-and-pour soap base
8 g sweet pea fragrance oil • 6 or 7 drops blue liquid colour
400 g opaque melt-and-pour soap base
10 g white musk fragrance oil

METHOD
Melt 300 g of the clear melt-and-pour soap base, add 6 g sweet pea fragrance oil and 2 or 3 drops of blue colouring. Pour a 1 cm layer into a tray mould. When set (about 15 minutes), remove from the tray and bend into a curl or swirl shape. Leave to set in the fridge (another 15 minutes). Melt another 200 g clear soap base, add 4 g white musk fragrance oil and 1 drop blue colouring. Pour a layer of about 0.5 cm in height into the tray mould. When set (allow 15 minutes), remove from the tray and bend into a curl or swirl shape. Leave to set in the fridge.

Melt the final 100g clear soap base with 100 g opaque soap base. Add 2 g sweet pea and 2 g white musk fragrance oils with another drop or two of blue liquid colouring. Pour a layer of about 0.5 cm in height into the tray mould. When set, remove from the tray and bend into a curl or swirl shape. Leave to set in the fridge.

Remove the three fragranced, blue swirls from the fridge and give them a spritz with isopropyl alcohol. Carefully place these swirls into an empty, washed and dried cylindrical cardboard tin such as the ones used to hold crisps. Melt the remaining 300 g opaque melt-and-pour soap base. When melted, add 4 g white musk fragrance oil and a drop or two of liquid blue colouring.

When the soap is cool enough, pour the soap over the swirls in the tin. Knock or tap the tin onto your work surface to remove any trapped air bubbles. Leave the soap to set.

To remove the soap from the tin, you will need to find where the outer cardboard wrapper meets the metal rim at the top of the tin. Using a pair of scissors, snip through the metal rim and carefully cut along the join and into the cardboard. Once you have cut enough that you can hold onto the cardboard, remove the scissors and peel away the tin by tearing down the join and unravelling the tin.

Cut the soap into slices.

Blue, blue soap

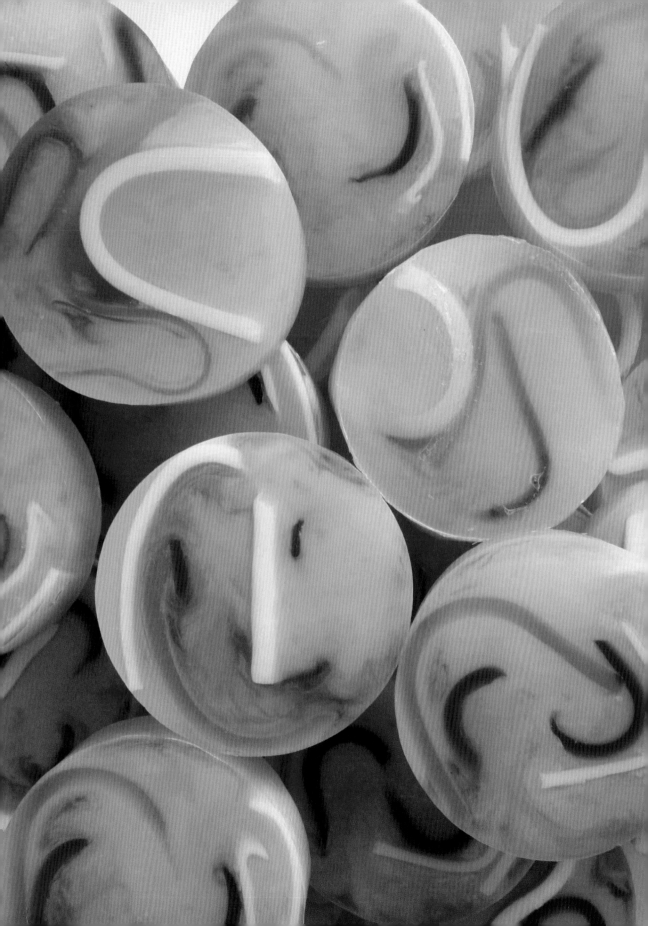

Girls just want to have fun soap

This soap reminds me of confetti and party streamers. It is also a great way of using up odd scraps of soap as you can melt the scraps and use them for the swirls and curls rather than starting with fresh soap base.

INGREDIENTS
900 g opaque melt-and-pour soap base
9 g jellybean fragrance oil
A few drops each of pink and blue liquid colour
9 g champagne fragrance oil

METHOD
Using 450g of the opaque soap base and the jellybean fragrance oil, make three sets of different colour swirls – one blue, one pink and the other either purple or a different shade of pink or blue. Put these in the fridge while you prepare the outer part of the soap loaf.

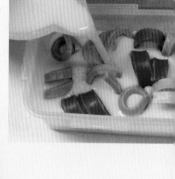

Pouring the white soap base over the soap curls

Melt the remaining 450 g of the opaque soap base and add 9 g champagne fragrance oil.

Place the coloured swirls and curls into the soap loaf mould and spritz with isopropyl alcohol. Making sure that the melted soap is cool enough to pour, but not so hot as to melt the swirls, carefully pour the soap over the curls and swirls until they are covered. Leave the soap loaf to set (about 15 minutes) before cutting into slices.

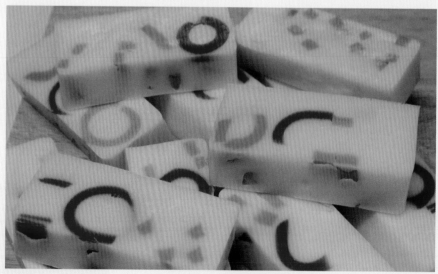

Curls and swirls embedded in white soap base

EMBEDDING PHOTOS IN SOAP

Personalised soaps make great gifts, promotional material or wedding favours.

Inspired by photographic cakes, where the cake is topped with an edible icing picture, our graphic soaps have given us hours of amusement. They are very simple to recreate – in fact the hardest part of the entire process is tracking down the special paper!

You will need printable A4 sheets of edible paper, such as wafer paper or rice paper (available from specialist cake decoration suppliers). To ensure your ink does not run when it gets wet, print using a laser printer rather than an inkjet printer.

Print your chosen design, logo or photograph onto the wafer or rice paper making sure that the printed output is the correct size for your soap mould. Carefully cut round the printed picture. Place a thin layer of clear melt-and-pour soap into your soap mould – the results are best if you do not use any colour and avoid using an essential or fragrance oil that may discolour or cloud the clear soap base.

Carefully place the photograph onto the soap – make sure you have it facing the right way up or down! You may get a better effect and more of an impact from the photograph if you leave a gap of about half a centimetre at the top of the mould. If you are using clear soap base for the whole bar, you can now carefully pour the rest of the soap base over the photograph, holding the photo in place with a cocktail stick to prevent it floating around. This soap base can be scented, if you wish.

Once your clear soap base has set (about 15 minutes), give it a spritz with isopropyl alcohol and then pour the final layer as an opaque layer (coloured or left white).

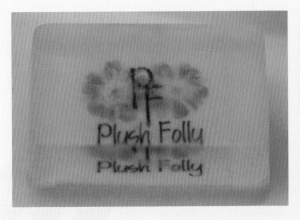

The Plush Folly logo printed on rice paper and embedded in soap

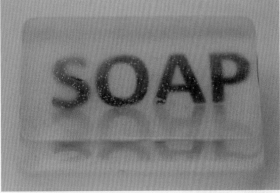

The 'soap' wording looks 3 dimensional

Making your own melt-and-pour soap base from scratch

Our friends at The Soap Kitchen (www.thesoapkitchen.co.uk) have perfected a recipe for melt-and-pour soap base and have very kindly permitted me to include it in this book. All the ingredients you will need can be sourced from The Soap Kitchen.

Like the traditional soap recipes, making your own melt-and-pour soap base involves the use of sodium hydroxide. This ingredient is considered hazardous unless handled correctly so please refer to the chapter on handling lye safely (pages 9–12). Once you have made the melt-and-pour soap base you can store it, cut it up, melt, fragrance, colour and shape it as you would any shop-bought melt-and-pour soap base. The soap made in the following recipe resembles the clear melt-and-pour soap base, but you can add titanium dioxide, a natural white colouring, to create a version of the opaque soap base.

Store the melt-and-pour soap base in an airtight container. If stored properly, the shelf life of your handmade melt-and-pour soap base will be at least three years.

EQUIPMENT NEEDED FOR MAKING MELT-AND-POUR SOAP BASE FROM SCRATCH

No specialist equipment is necessary and quite possibly you will already have everything you need. Key pieces of equipment include:

- Heatproof jug(s)
- Large stainless steel saucepan
- Stainless steel spoons for stirring
- A set of digital scales to weigh the ingredients
- Plastic or silicone container as the soap mould
- Safety equipment (goggles and gloves)

Melt-and-pour soap making ingredients with the finished soap

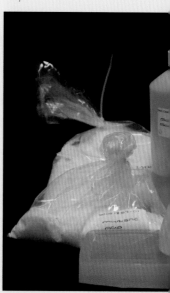

HOW TO MAKE MELT-AND-POUR SOAP BASE

To make white melt-and-pour soap base, add a little titanium dioxide to the melted soap base.

Prepare your ingredients in the following groups.

PHASE 1 – LYE

67.5 g cold tap water • 67.5 g sodium hydroxide

PHASE 2 – BASE INGREDIENTS

422.5 g mono propylene glycol • 162.5 g glycerine
443.5 g sorbitol solution (70 per cent)
675 g sodium C14/C16 olefin sulphonate

PHASE 3 – FATTY ACIDS

295 g stearic acid • 137.5 g myristic acid

PHASE 4 – FINAL PHASE

22.5 g myristic acid • 59 g triethanolamine

METHOD

Phase 1 – Making sure you pay careful attention to the lye safety guidelines (pages 9 and 10), weigh the water and place it in a heatproof jug. Weigh the sodium hydroxide and carefully tip it into the water. Stir the lye well until all the grainy pieces have dissolved. Set aside.

Phase 2 – Weigh all the Phase 2 ingredients and place them in a large saucepan. You will be making nearly 2.5 kg of soap base so the saucepan must be large enough to accommodate at least 3 litres. Heat, stirring constantly, until a temperature of 60°C (140°F) is reached. A sugar thermometer would be perfect for checking this.

Phase 3 – When the temperature has reached 60°C (140°F) add the Phase 3 ingredients and stir well. Increase to 74°C (165°F).

Phase 4 – Once the temperature has reached 74°C (165°F), slowly add the lye solution and stir gently for two to three minutes (do not stir too vigorously or you will create a froth). Leave on the hob over a low to medium heat for up to 20 minutes, stirring every four or five minutes until the soap mixture has turned completely transparent.

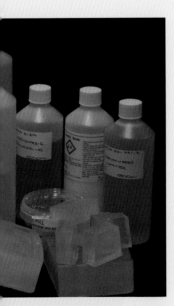

Place a lid on the saucepan and leave on a low to medium heat for one hour without stirring. You should aim to have the soap mixture at a constant 74°C (165°F).

After one hour, add the final batch of ingredients and stir until melted. Remove the saucepan from the heat and cool slightly. When the mixture has cooled to 65°C (149°F), pour into moulds and leave to set.

When the soap base has cooled and hardened, remove it from the moulds and treat as you would the regular melt-and-pour soap base.

CHAPTER FIVE

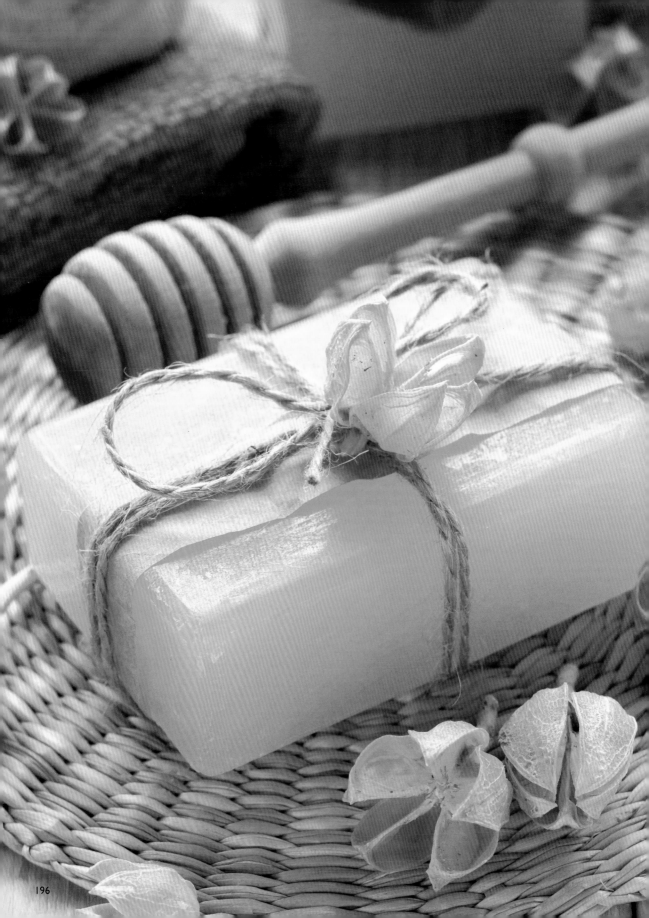

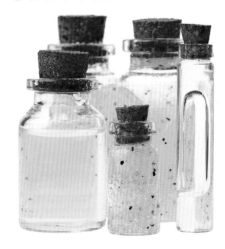

Using surfactants

Liquid soap products can be made using premade bases called surfactants. Unlike melt-and-pour soap base, the surfactants need to be added to other ingredients in order for you to create a finished, useable product. They will also need preserving in order to have a shelf life beyond a week or so.

Surfactants are made by processing oils and their fatty acids to create an undiluted soap base. This is exactly what you would do if you were making liquid soap, since that method involves processing the oils with potassium hydroxide to create a paste, which then needs diluting further. The technical name for the paste is potassium cocoate, potassium olivate, potassium castorate or similar depending on the base oils used.

Using a surfactant to make your liquid soaps cuts out the lye creation stage, which some people prefer to avoid since they are nervous about handling the potassium hydroxide. You will be starting with ingredients such as sodium cocoyl isethionate and cocoglucoside rather than creating these yourself.

What are surfactants?

The word surfactant is short for 'surface active agent' meaning that a surfactant interacts with the surface of a liquid to change its properties. A surfactant has a hydrophilic (water-loving) head and a lipophilic (oil-loving) or hydrophobic (water-hating) tail. All surfactants are partly water-soluble and partly oil-soluble. This allows oils and waters, which normally don't mix together, to combine. A surfactant is often referred to as a wetting agent. There is a wide range of surfactants available and whilst they all do the same job (clean!), they have different textures (thick liquid, granules, fine powder, etc.). Surfactants work through a process known as 'adsorption', which means that they accumulate on the surface of water or other liquid, creating a film that reduces surface tension. For example, soap (which is also a surfactant) is used to break the surface tension of water so that it can penetrate more fully. The foaming action of soap helps water get under dirt, grime and grease on surfaces such as your skin, dishes and clothes, allowing the water to carry the dirt away. If you try to wash your hands without soap the high surface tension of non-soapy water makes it very difficult to remove dirt.

Formulating with surfactants

When designing your liquid soap using surfactants you'll need to decide how concentrated you want the liquid soap product to be. Often the surfactant content is as much as 50 per cent with the remaining 50 per cent being water or a combination of water and other ingredients to give the soap a smell, preserve and thicken it, add colour and so on. But you don't have to use 50 per cent and it is perfectly acceptable to make a liquid soap using only 20–40 per cent surfactants with the rest water and other ingredients.

Some surfactants are known for their highly effective cleaning ability but these can also be drying on the skin. Others are very mild and suitable for sensitive skins, but don't create much lather. Some surfactants create an abundance of bubbles but can cause skin dryness. It's all a matter of understanding what does what and how they can work together to create the perfect product for you.

The perfect bubble bath product demands a large proportion of a high foaming surfactant, whilst the perfect shampoo will have good cleansing properties, high foaming properties, as well as being mild and gentle. Facial cleansers will need to be mild and have limited foaming ability.

Considering there are well over 100 different surfactants available on the market, to cover them all is another book in itself so I will discuss only a handful here. Those that I have selected are available from cosmetic ingredient suppliers whose contact details can be found on page 207.

USING GLUCOSIDES

The glucoside range of surfactants is produced from renewable raw materials including corn sugar and coconut oil fatty acids. They are biodegradable, mild and gentle, with good foaming ability.

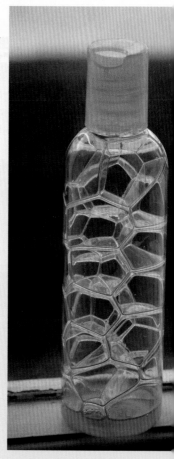

Surfactants can be used to create quick and easy foaming liquid soap products

There are three main surfactants in the glucoside family. These are coco glucoside, lauryl glucoside and decyl glucoside. The coco and lauryl glucosides are thick, clear liquids whilst the lauryl glucoside is a thick, white sticky paste. Each of these glucosides can be used at up to 50 per cent, meaning they can form at least half of your recipe. The glucosides produce a thin product that is likely to need thickening up.

USING COCAMIDOPROPYL BETAINE

Cocamidopropyl betaine is a mild surfactant with fairly good foaming abilities. It tends to be used with other surfactants that have better foaming abilities as it can make the overall product a lot milder.

Cocamidopropyl betaine is a thin, clear liquid and often used with the thicker surfactants to make them more manageable. It can form up to 40 per cent of your final liquid soap product.

USING SODIUM COCOYL ISETHIONATE

Sodium cocoyl isethionate is a white powder that needs to be carefully dissolved in water before it can be applied to the skin. It is very mild and foams up well. Whilst it doesn't have deep cleansing abilities, it makes a very lovely body wash.

Sodium cocoyl isethionate will create a very thick product and needs only to be used at up to 16 per cent. It is prone to making the product runnier when warm (and thicker, when cold) and can change viscosity in hot or cold bathrooms.

Surfactant recipes

Making a liquid soap product with surfactants is relatively quick and easy; it is also much quicker than making liquid soap from scratch. Whilst making surfactant products may not be difficult, it can be quite tricky getting the correct thickness since some surfactants remain very fluid until they are cold, whilst others are very thick to start off with. The good news is that if your final product is too thick, you can always add a little more water to make it slightly runnier. Each of these recipes makes 200 g of liquid soap.

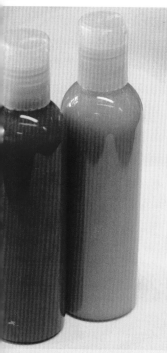

Mica can be used to add colour and shimmer to surfactant soaps

THICKENING YOUR LIQUID SOAP

If your final product is too thin, you can thicken it up by adding up to 2 per cent gum (such as xanthan or guar) and leaving the gum to dissolve and thicken. Alternatively, you can add table salt. Start with 5 per cent salt and stir well. Keep adding a little more until you have reached the desired thickness. Note that not all fragrance and essential oils work with salt and may cause the liquid soap to separate.

After adding your thickening agent it is sensible to leave the product for a few hours to adjust to its final viscosity. During this time it may become thicker to the point of becoming too thick and will then require a little watering down. The ambient temperature, the amount of agitation and stirring plus the format of the surfactant all have an impact on the final viscosity so don't be surprised if you have a product that works well in the winter but is a little too runny when you make it again during the summer. A foamer pump is a special pump bottle that will dispense a handful of foam rather than liquid soap. If you are using foamer bottles the liquid soap needs to be thin in order for it to be pumped into the foaming mechanism.

Mild and gentle body wash

So mild and gentle that it is suitable for even the most sensitive of skins. That said, I've scented this version with a current favourite of mine: blood orange. It might not suit everyone's skin or taste so feel free to substitute it with whatever aroma suits you.

INGREDIENTS
40 g coco glucoside • 40 g lauryl glucoside • 20 g decyl glucoside
2 g xanthan gum • 100 g hot spring water • 10 g d-panthenol
4 g blood orange essential oil • 2 g GFphen PCG preservative
A pinch of autumn red mica colour • 2–10 g table salt

METHOD
Weigh the glucosides and gum into a heatproof bowl or jug. Pour over the hot spring water and stir well.

Leave the mixture to cool a little before adding the d-panthenol and stir again. The xanthan gum takes a while to dissolve and will make your product look a little speckly until then. To speed up the process, you can use a small whisk or milk frother to break down the xanthan particles otherwise time and gentle stirring or squashing will suffice.

Add the blood orange essential oil, preservative and a pinch of mica and stir again. Leave to cool completely before deciding whether the product requires additional thickening (add more gum or up to 5 per cent salt) or thinning (add a little hot water).

Place the liquid soap in the bottle when the product is cool and at the correct thickness. It will keep for up to nine months.

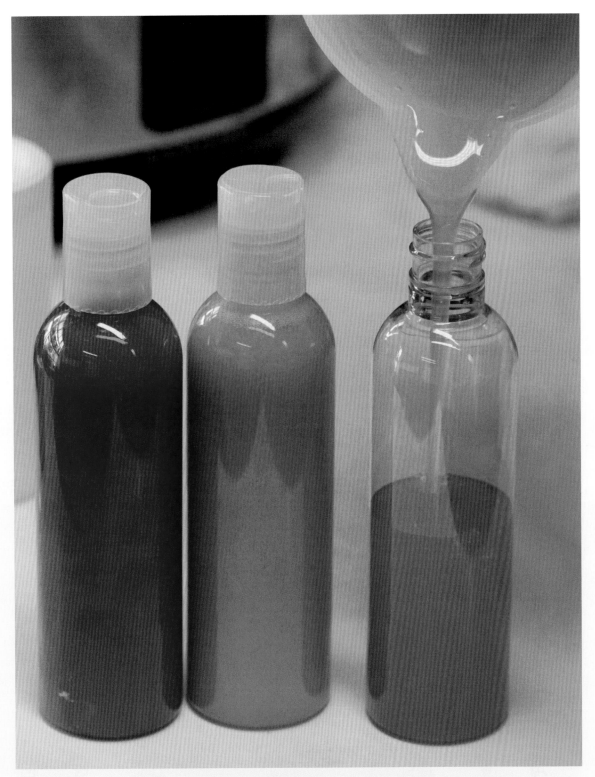

Mild and gentle body wash and Pure opulence Midas bathing wash

Wake-up shower cream

Lively and uplifting bergamot and pink grapefruit will certainly energise and get you going for the day!

This liquid soap is made with sodium cocoyl isethionate, which slowly turns from clear to opaque as it cools and thickens. It can be difficult to dissolve so don't be tempted to stir until you have left it sitting in hot water for at least five minutes. Make sure every bit of the sodium cocoyl isethionate has dissolved – you may find this easier if you heat the product up over a gentle heat.

Ingredients
20 g sodium cocoyl isethionate • 140 g hot spring water
22 g cocamidopropyl betaine • 10 g d-panthenol
2 g bergamot essential oil • 2 g pink grapefruit essential oil
2 g GFphen PCG preservative • 1 drop pink liquid colour
8–10 g table salt or 2 g xanthan gum, if necessary (see below)

Method
Weigh the sodium cocoyl isethionate into a heatproof bowl or jug. Pour over the hot spring water and leave to seep for at least five minutes. Do not be tempted to stir during this time.

After five minutes you can stir the sodium cocoyl isethionate into the water. Make sure that every bit is dissolved. If necessary, warm it up to facilitate the dissolving process.

Once the sodium cocoyl isethionate has dissolved, add the cocamidopropyl betaine and d-panthenol; stir again.

Add the bergamot and pink grapefruit essential oils, preservative and liquid colouring; stir again. Leave to cool at room temperature, preferably for at least 24 hours.

If you are happy with the thickness of the product after 24 hours, place it in the bottle. However if it is a little on the thick side, add a small amount of hot water and stir it into the product. Do not be surprised if the product goes thin again. If it does, just leave for a further 24 hours to thicken up before transferring it to the bottle.

If it is on the thin side, add up to 10 g salt or up to 2 g xanthan gum. Stir well and leave for a few hours to settle to its final viscosity.

Pure opulence Midas bathing wash

This recipe contains additional glycerine to add glide and bubbles to the soap. I've also included a little gold mica just to give a slight gold colour. If you like floral smells but haven't experienced champaca before, you'll wonder how you've ever managed without it – truly glorious!

INGREDIENTS
20 g sodium cocoyl isethionate • 100 g hot spring water
50 g warmed aloe vera • 26 g coco glucoside • 10 g d-panthenol
18 g glycerine • 4 g champaca fragrance oil
2 g GFphen PCG preservative • 6–10 g table salt
$^1/_2$ teaspoon gold mica

METHOD
Weigh the sodium cocoyl isethionate into a heatproof bowl or jug. Pour over the hot spring water and leave to seep for at least five minutes (do not be tempted to stir during this time).

After five minutes add the warmed aloe vera and stir. Make sure that every bit of sodium cocoyl isethionate has dissolved. If necessary, warm it up and stir to facilitate the dissolving process.

Once the sodium cocoyl isethionate has dissolved, add the coco glucoside, d-panthenol and glycerine; stir again.

Add the champaca (inhale its beautiful aroma as you pour!) and the preservative; stir well. Leave to cool at room temperature, preferably for at least 24 hours.

Adjust the viscosity by adding salt and stir again, giving the mixture a chance to settle. When the product has naturally thickened up, add the gold mica and gently stir it into the soap. Transfer to a bottle.

Energise pre-party body wash

Geranium, black pepper and juniper berry will certainly energise and get you in a party mood!

Ingredients
15 g sodium cocoyl isetheionate • 140 g hot water
20 g coco glucoside • 20 g glycerine
2 g GFphen PCG preservative • 1 g geranium essential oil
0.5 g black pepper essential oil • 0.5 g juniper berry essential oil
4–8 g salt

Method
Place the sodium cocoyl isetheionate in a large saucepan and pour over the hot water. Add the coco glucoside and glycerine but do not stir immediately. Leave to seep for five minutes and then stir. If the sodium cocoyl isethionate does not dissolve into the hot water, place over a gentle heat and stir gently until it has fully dissolved.

Off the heat, add the preservative and essential oils and stir again. Add 4 g salt and stir again. Leave to cool and thicken before decanting (the preservative means it will last for up to a year).

Making non-lye melt-and-pour soap from scratch

And finally… In my experiments with surfactants I challenged myself to make a hard bar of soap from scratch but without using sodium hydroxide at all. After several attempts (some were too soft, others didn't foam up sufficiently), I made a batch of creamy, moisturising, hard, white bars of soap. The recipe below is for one bar of soap only.

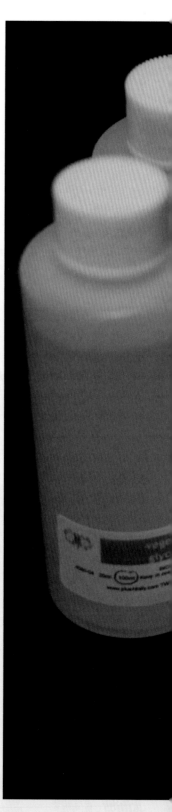

Sal's creamy white soap challenge

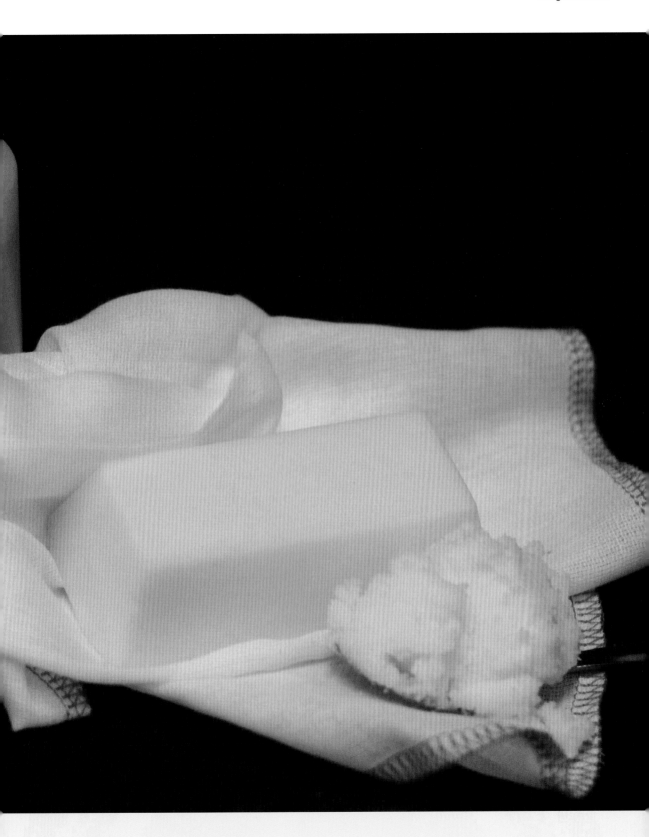

Sal's creamy white soap challenge

INGREDIENTS
50 g sodium cocoyl isethionate • 16 g coco glucoside
10 g stearic acid • 10 g shea butter
7 g emulsifying wax • 3 g d-panthenol
2 g soft almond fragrance oil

METHOD
Weigh the sodium cocoyl isethionate, coco glucoside, stearic acid, shea butter and emulsifying wax into a heatproof bowl or jug. Heat until the stearic acid has melted and the mixture has become quite soft. Note that the mixture won't be completely fluid, but it must be soft and pliable without any signs of graininess.

Remove from the heat and quickly stir in the d-panthenol and fragrance oil (you need to work quickly as the mixture will want to start setting). Dollop the soap into the mould and bang the mould onto the work surface to smooth out the surface and remove any air bubbles. I found I got a smoother finish if I popped the soap into the fridge straightaway. As soon as the soap has cooled and set hard it is ready for use.

Resources

All of the ingredients, packaging and specialist equipment needed to make the different soaps outlined in this book can be purchased online. Do keep an eye out for many of the ingredients in your local supermarket, too, as lots of the oils and decorations are also used in cooking.

ESSENTIAL OILS

Freshskin www.freshskin.co.uk Tel: 07846 174876
id Aromatics www.idaromatics.co.uk Tel: 0113 242 4983

INGREDIENTS AND PACKAGING

Gracefruit Limited www.gracefruit.com Tel: 01324 841353
Shea Butter Cottage www.sheabuttercottage.co.uk Tel: 020 8144 4609
Soap Basics www.soapbasics.co.uk Tel: 01225 899286
The Soap Kitchen www.thesoapkitchen.co.uk Tel: 01805 622944
Summer Naturals www.summernaturals.co.uk

MOULDS

DennyCraft Moulds www.dennycraftmoulds.co.uk Tel: 01262 604819
The Moulds Shop www.themouldsshop.co.uk

PHOTOGRAPHS

Lizzi Roche Photography www.facebook.com/LizziRochePhotography
Tom Weller Photography www.tomwellerphotography.com Tel: 07986 071970

SPECIALIST HERBS, GUMS AND RESINS

G. Baldwin & Co www.baldwins.co.uk Tel: 020 7703 5550
The Organic Herb Trading Co www.organicherbtrading.com Tel: 01823 401205

TRAINING COURSES, KITS, INGREDIENTS AND PACKAGING

Plush Folly www.plushfolly.com Tel: 020 3002 2507

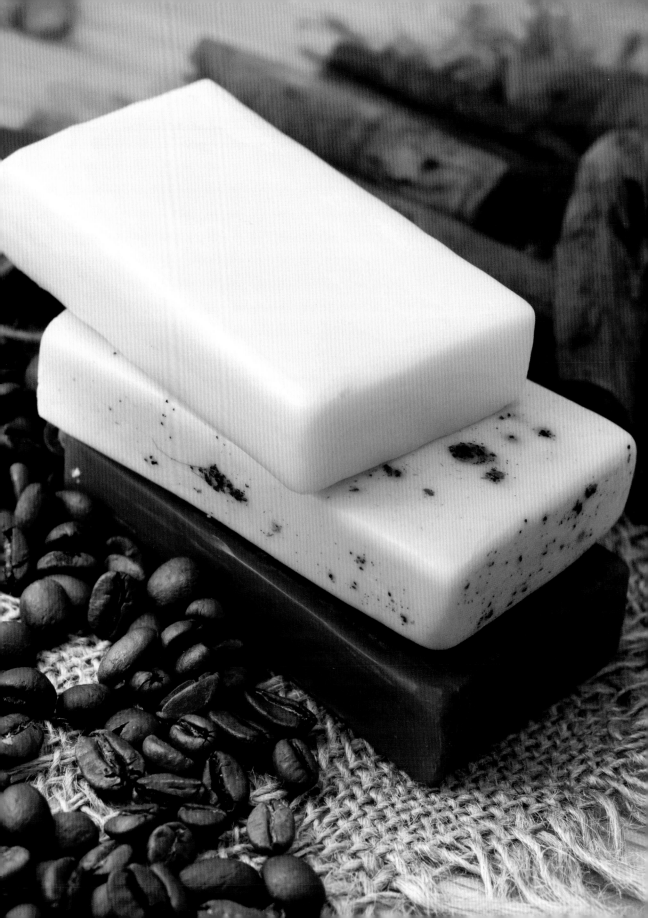

Index